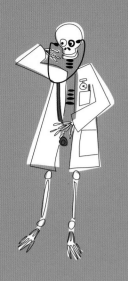

Flesh and Bones of
ANATOMY

Susie Whiten MA PhD

Senior Lecturer
Bute Medical School
University of St Andrews
St Andrews
UK

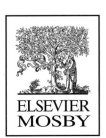

ELSEVIER
MOSBY

Edinburgh   London   New York   Oxford   Philadelphia   St Louis   Sydney   Toronto   2006

ELSEVIER
MOSBY

1005081 721

First published 2006

ISBN-13: 978 07234 33545
ISBN-10: 07234 33542

British Library Cataloguing in Publication Data
A catalogue record for this book is available from the British Library

Library of Congress Cataloging in Publication Data
A catalog record for this book is available from the Library of Congress

Notice
Neither the Publisher nor the Author assume any responsibility for any loss or injury and/or damage to persons or property arising out of or related to any use of the material contained in this book. It is the responsibility of the treating practitioner, relying on independent expertise and knowledge of the patient, to determine the best treatment and method of application for the patient.
The Publisher

Printed in China

The publisher's policy is to use **paper manufactured from sustainable forests**

Working together to grow
libraries in developing countries

www.elsevier.com | www.bookaid.org | www.sabre.org

ELSEVIER | BOOK AID International | Sabre Foundation

your source for books, journals and multimedia in the health sciences

www.elsevierhealth.com

Flesh and Bones of
ANATOMY

Commissioning Editor: **Timothy Horne**
Development Editors: **Barbara Simmons, Jane Ward**
Project Manager: **Frances Affleck**
Designer: **Jayne Jones**
Illustrator: **Jenni Miller**

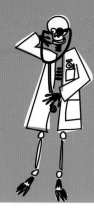

Contents

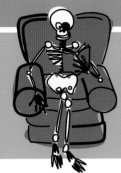

The big picture

The complex structures of the human body is truly awesome and a source of never ending fascination for many people. Learning anatomy and understanding how the structure of the body relates to its functions has been the foundation of medical education and practice for hundreds of years. Medical students gradually build up their knowledge of the body, eventually becoming experts who can apply their knowledge to solve novel clinical problems. You will need to know your anatomy well to be able to examine your patients effectively, to recognize abnormality and to perform procedures safely. Your aim must be to have an accurate, three-dimensional image of the body in your head.

Historically, medical students learnt anatomy by literally taking a body apart. In recent times, this approach has been questioned and students may be expected to know their way around the body using different strategies based on modern technology. Modern medical imaging techniques and the wide availability of quite stunning digital images of the body have revolutionized teaching and learning. It is hard to say what is the *best* method of learning anatomy (and individual students differ anyway), but all are agreed about the outcome. Putting it simply, a medical practitioner must have X-ray vision! When examining a patient or performing a clinical procedure, doctors must have in mind a three-dimensional image of what lies beneath the skin. In addition, they should be aware of the range of normal variation both between individuals and within the same individual at different times of their life; an understanding of normal structure is important because *your job is to be able to recognize abnormality.*

HOW TO LEARN ANATOMY

Historically, anatomy has involved naming and classifying structures but always with an underlying curiosity about how they function and how to explain what is happening when disease changes the structure. Modern anatomy that is relevant to your professional training is functional anatomy. There are three ways of organizing the study of anatomy: systematic, regional and clinical.

Systematic anatomy is a sequential study of the functional systems of the body. It is usually how anatomy is tackled in integrated medical curricula. It often does make sense to group structures that work together to perform a particular function because they will share common physiological mechanisms (e.g. cardiovascular system) and some have physiological effects across the entire body (e.g. nervous and endocrine systems).

Regional anatomy recognizes that the body is organized into specific parts (regions such as thorax, head and neck, and the limbs). The major regions are subdivided to ease understanding.

Regional anatomy takes into account the arrangement and relationships of adjacent organs from different systems. Knowledge of the regional organization is useful when performing a physical examination and may be vital in treatment; for example, if a patient is stabbed in the abdomen, it might simultaneously affect the digestive, urinary and cardiovascular systems. In the same way, a tumour in the thorax may affect a number of structures from several different systems. The regional approach is often used when studying anatomy by dissection.

Clinical anatomy is the application of anatomy to the symptoms experienced by patients. Students cheerfully learn the action of a muscle and may be able to give correct responses to questions such as 'what are the flexors of the elbow joint?'. However, can you answer the applied question. 'How would a patient present if the flexors of his elbow were paralysed?' 'What tests would you perform to confirm your diagnosis?'

There is a lot of anatomy and it is often hard to know where to start and what to focus on. Just how much should a student know? The big picture discusses some general principles that may help to answer this. Here is some very general advice.

Learn about big things first.   It will sometimes seem as if anatomy is made up of endless layers of detail. Take a broad view before you begin to tackle the details. For example, the blood supply of the heart is a very important topic; obviously it is essential to learn about the coronary arteries and what they supply. However, the arteries are described in textbooks *in relation to the structure of the heart* and so it is sensible to start by learning the orientation of the heart, the names of its surfaces and which chambers make up those surfaces before attempting to read about the detailed course and distribution of the coronary arteries.

Learn anatomy slowly.   It really is impossible to cram (and understand) it in just a few sessions.

Start with the bones.   For each of the regions, start with the bones and, if possible, have the individual bones in your hand as you learn. *You need to know how a bone articulates with others, the major markings and what attaches to them.*

Use your own body. You can learn surface anatomy and important landmarks; these are common to all of us (they can't take that away from you!).

Once you have learned the basics of adult anatomy, explore some **embryology**; it often really helps in understanding complicated structures like the gut and will certainly explain congenital abnormality.

Read through this section before you start and again when you have tackled some of the anatomy. It gives an overview of some important aspects of regional anatomy and then looks at some of the systems that have relevance across regions (e.g. the nervous system). Some aspects will seem difficult but knowledge of general principles will help you to make the links that lead to real understanding.

■ THE BODY WALL AND TRUNK

The body is divided into the trunk, the limbs and the head and neck. The trunk consists of the body wall enclosing serous cavities that contain the organs of the body (viscera). The thorax is separated from the abdomen by the diaphragm; inferiorly, the pelvic diaphragm separates the pelvic contents from the perineum.

The close anatomical relationships in the thorax, abdomen and pelvis mean that disease in one system will affect others very rapidly and can lead to complex and confusing symptoms.

You must learn the anatomy of the body wall, the position of all the viscera in relation to one another and to their surface land-marks because it is essential for:

- physical examination of the major systems (cardiovascular, respiratory, digestive, etc.)
- interpretation of radiographs
- understanding computed tomographic and magnetic resonance scans
- relating the position of major structures to their **vertebral levels** (Table 1.1 and Fig. 3.1.3).

The general structure of the body wall follows the same pattern whether in the thorax, abdomen or pelvis and perineum. There are three muscle layers. The nerves, arteries and veins are organized segmentally and lie between the middle and deepest layers of muscle in the **neurovascular plane**.

The nerve supply is from spinal nerves (p. 30). The **dorsal rami** supply the erector spinae muscles and skin of the back. The **ventral rami** supply the lateral and anterior muscles and skin. The blood supply of the body wall arises from posterior and anterior arteries, linked by anastomoses. Posteriorly, the body wall is supplied by lateral segmental branches of the aorta (intercostal and lumbar arteries). The anterior wall is supplied by branches of the subclavian and external iliac arteries (internal thoracic, superior

and inferior epigastric arteries; p. 82). Segmental veins drain the posterior body wall and unite to form the **azygos** and **hemiazygos veins** (see p. 69). They, in turn, are also connected with the vertebral venous plexus that surrounds the spinal cord; this link explains the spread of cancer from thoracic and pelvic viscera to vertebral bodies.

Serous cavities

Some organs are relatively mobile (e.g. heart, stomach) and their surfaces come into contact with other viscera and with the body wall. To reduce friction and allow free movement of the viscera, the body cavities and organs are lined by smooth, moist membranes:

- the lungs are enclosed by pleural membranes, which line the pleural cavity
- the heart is surrounded by the pericardium, which lines the pericardial cavity
- the abdominal viscera are covered by the peritoneum, which lines the peritoneal cavity.

The outer part of the membrane is known as the parietal layer and the part that covers the organs is the visceral layer; a serous fluid is secreted into the intervening space (Fig. 1.1 and p. 58). Some abdominal organs are particularly mobile because they are suspended by folds of peritoneum known as **mesenteries** (p. 80). Mesenteries carry blood vessels and lymphatics between the body wall to the viscera.

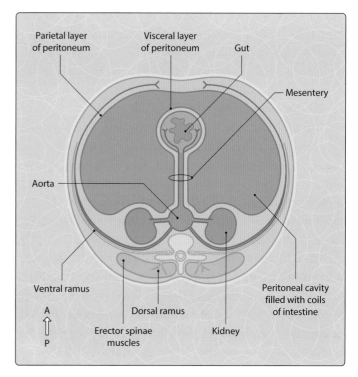

Fig. 1.1 Transverse section through the trunk to show the general plan of the posterior abdominal wall, the layers of the peritoneum and the formation of the gut mesentery with its blood supply.

Table 1.1 SUMMARY OF VERTEBRAL LEVELS

Position	Structure	Vertebral level
Hyoid bone	Tonsillar node	C2
Superior border of the thyroid cartilage	Bifurcation of the common carotid artery	C3
Thyroid prominence	Vocal fold	C4
Cricothyroid membrane	Site of laryngotomy	C5
Cricoid cartilage	Beginning of trachea and oesophagus	C6
Vertebra prominens		C7
Sternoclavicular joints	Formation of brachiocephalic veins. Bifurcation of the brachiocephalic trunk	T1, T2
Jugular or suprasternal notch (midline)	Trachea; highest point of the arch of the aorta	T2
	Brachiocephalic veins unite to form superior vena cava	T3
Sternal angle (of Louis) (intercostal cartilage)	Lower limit of the arch of the aorta; bifurcation of the trachea; aortic impression on oesophagus; arch of azygos vein	T4
	Hilum of the lung; left main bronchus impression on oesophagus	T5/6
Nipple/4th intercostal space		T7
7th intercostal cartilage	Caval opening in the diaphragm	T8
5th intercostal cartilage	Apex heart beat	
Xiphoid process	Oesophageal opening in the diaphragm	T10
Ribs 9, 10 and 11	Spleen	T11 (approximately)
Rib 12	Aorta, thoracic duct and azygos and hemiazygos veins pass through the aortic hiatus of the diaphragm; origin of the coeliac trunk from the aorta; upper pole of the kidneys; costodiaphragmatic recess	T12
	Origin of the superior mesenteric artery from the aorta	T12/ L1
Transpyloric plane: tip of the 9th costal cartilage	Origin of the superior mesenteric artery; gall bladder; pylorus; duodenojejunal flexure; hilum of the kidneys; head of the pancreas	L1
Subcostal plane	Origin of the gonadal and inferior mesenteric arteries	L2/3
Umbilicus	Bifurcation of the aorta (below and left)	L3/4
Line between the iliac crests	Lumbar puncture; epidural anaesthesia	L3/4
Anterior superior iliac spine	Attachment of the inguinal ligament	L5

Thorax

The *embryological development of the thoracic viscera* has important influences on postnatal anatomy. The heart and developing diaphragm arise in the cervical region of the embryo, acquiring their nerve and blood supply at a very early stage. Later developmental events cause the heart and diaphragm to shift towards the thoracic region and the viscera carry their original innervation to this new location. Consequently, the heart receives sympathetic nerve fibres from the *cervical sympathetic ganglia*; the phrenic nerves that supply the pericardium, pleura, diaphragm and diaphragmatic peritoneum are branches of the *cervical plexus* (C_3, C_4, C_5). The *cervical innervation of the diaphragm* is very important. A patient sustaining a cervical fracture that damages the spinal cord at C_3 will be unable to breathe unaided and may die (C_3, C_4, C_5 keep the diaphragm, and the patient, alive).

Abdomen

The embryological development of the gut tube is very helpful in understanding the arrangement of the viscera, their peritoneal attachments and congenital abnormalities (p. 80). The whole of the embryonic gut tube is suspended from the posterior wall by the dorsal mesentery. Only the foregut and its outgrowths are also attached to the anterior wall by a ventral mesentery. Consequently, the ventral mesentery has a free edge just below the liver in which the bile duct develops (Fig. 3.28.1). As the gut develops, it undergoes dramatic changes of position, creating complex folds of mesentery and resulting in the formation of folds and recesses such as the lesser sac, hepatorenal and subphrenic spaces. These spaces may be the sites of accumulation of pus or blood.

The anterior abdominal wall is so often inspected, palpated and incised surgically that it is important to learn its anatomy and how to describe the different quadrants (p. 76). If you understand how the testes develop in the abdomen and descend to the scrotum you will be able to understand the origin of their blood supply, the route of their lymphatic drainage and the anatomy of inguinal hernia.

The integrity of the pelvic diaphragm, which separates the pelvic contents from the perineum, is important in the context of faecal continence and support of the uterus. You should also understand the anatomy of urinary continence. Loss of control will be devastating for the individual. There are clinically important transitional zones in the anal canal and at the external os of the uterine cervix where there is a developmental boundary between external body wall and internal visceral structures. Remember that the blood supply, venous and lymphatic drainage and innervation all reflect this inside/outside watershed.

THE LIMBS

It can be surprising to see that the arrangement of bones in the limbs of a dinosaur is strikingly similar to other vertebrate limbs including our own; the pentadactyl (five-fingered) limb is an ancient pattern. Human upper and lower limbs are based on this plan and are modified for different aspects of locomotion. Our tree-dwelling primate ancestors developed highly mobile forelimbs for climbing and grasping. Our more recent forebears became increasingly bipedal. These mechanical requirements have resulted in specific modifications of the basic pattern.

The limbs are attached to the trunk through the pelvic and pectoral girdles. The **pelvic girdle** is a rigid ring of bone, firmly attached to the vertebral column to transmit forces from the powerful limb muscles. However, the **pectoral girdle** consists of the clavicles and scapula and is an incomplete ring; the only bony attachment is through the sternoclavicular joint. In fact, the upper limb is mainly attached by powerful muscles at the root of the limb, which dramatically increases its overall mobility.

However, both limbs have a similar arrangement of joints: a proximal ball and socket (hip and shoulder), a hinge (knee and elbow) a further joint that allows rotation (complex joints at the ankle and wrist) and a series of multiple hinge joints (toes and fingers).

The deep fascia of the limbs form a sleeve (or stocking) around the muscles and the neurovascular bundles that supply them. Septa arise from the tubes of fascia and are attached deeply to bone, more or less separating groups of muscles into compartments in which muscles share a common function and nerve supply. *The arrangement of fascia is important in the limbs.* It allows muscles to contract independently and controls how blood or infection may spread. In the lower limb, the tube of deep fascia surrounding the leg is part of the mechanism that brings about the return of venous blood to the heart (p. 109).

The development of varicose veins and of compartment syndrome both relate to the organization of the deep fascia.

Upper limb

Like our ability to talk, our hands and what we can do with them are unique in the animal kingdom. It is not an exaggeration to say that the ability to oppose the thumb with our fingers has enabled us to make and manipulate the tools that have underpinned human cultural evolution.

The human hand is a versatile grasping organ at the end of a series of jointed levers. The role of the proximal muscles acting on the shoulder is to manoeuvre the hand into its various working positions literally anywhere in the space around our bodies. The distal flexor muscles of the forearm act on the joints of the hand to allow it to perform a multitude of functions ranging from the **power grip** required to carry a heavy bag of shopping or grip a hammer to the delicate **pinch grip** required to pick up a needle or use a keyboard. The skin of the hand is also exquisitely sensitive; try using a mobile phone wearing gloves! You will appreciate that upper limb injuries, particularly hand injuries, are very disabling and can be devastating for a patient.

The upper limb is frequently damaged in falls on the outstretched hand. The glenohumeral joint is the most commonly dislocated large joint; the clavicle is the most commonly fractured bone, and one in four patients visiting accident and emergency departments is suffering from a hand injury. The axillary, radial and ulnar nerves lie in direct contact with the humerus and are vulnerable to damage.

In the arm and forearm, deep fascia divides the muscles into anterior, flexor (supplied by the median and ulnar nerves) and posterior extensor compartments (supplied by the radial nerve). The intrinsic muscles of the hand are supplied by the ulnar nerve except for the important short muscles of the thumb and the lateral two lumbricals, which are innervated by the median nerve.

Lower limb

Some would argue that, because we are bipedal, the foot is more highly evolved than the hand. While we are upright, the feet must balance our *entire* body weight whether we are standing still or moving in some way. Moreover, we do it apparently without effort or sense of weight.

The powerful muscles and joints of the lower limbs move the whole body relative to the ground as we walk and move the free limb on the trunk (e.g. kicking a ball). The muscles of the lower limbs also have an important function in allowing us just to remain upright. In a normal standing position, the line of gravity falls behind the hip and in front of the knee and ankle joints. We continually make subtle postural adjustments to prevent ourselves either from falling backwards at our hips or forwards over our knees and ankles. The force of gravity influences the position and strength of the muscles and ligaments that support the lower limb joints.

The joints of the lower limb are stable when we stand upright. The tarsals are altogether more massive than the carpal bones because they carry all the body weight. The talus distributes the weight through medial and longitudinal arches to the other bones of the foot. Sprained ankle is one of the commonest injuries in everyday life and *all* the joints of the lower limb are vulnerable to damage in sporting activities.

An important difference between the upper and lower limbs arises during embryonic development, when the lower limb rotates medially. This explains why:

- the extensors of the knee lie on the *front* of the thigh while the flexors lie *behind* (compare it with the arm where the flexors of the elbow are anterior and the extensors posterior)
- the knee points forwards (the elbow points backwards)
- the sole of the foot is equivalent to the palm of the hand
- the dermatomes of the lower limb spiral down the limb
- the main arterial stem follows a spiral around the femur.

The roots of the sciatic nerve may be compressed by a prolapsed intervertebral disc in the lumbar region, giving rise to sciatica. However, the nerve most vulnerable to direct damage is the **common peroneal nerve** as it passes around the neck of the fibula. Damage results in 'foot drop'.

The pattern of venous drainage is important in the lower limb as the valves of large, superficial veins are prone to damage, resulting in the development of varicose veins.

■ HEAD AND NECK

The anatomy of the head and neck is complex and really fascinating. I warn you that you are unlikely to pull it together until you have completed your first overview of the region.

The skull houses the brain and special senses and it supports the beginning of the respiratory and digestive tracts; when it is damaged, the results can be very serious indeed. Structures within the skull are intimately related and disease can spread rapidly, causing multisystem problems. Think of the skull in three parts:

- **facial bones**: several irregular-shaped bones forming a wedge shape tucked under the cranium; they are fragile and easily fractured
- **cranium**: several thin flat bones articulating at immovable joints form a strong protective brain box
- **mandible**: articulates with part of the temporal bone to form the temporomandibular joint.

Begin by learning the arrangement of the bones of the skull.

There are numerous holes through which structures pass (**foramina**); as you study the major foramina, you should learn what structures pass through them (many carry cranial nerves). Head and neck anatomy is really the functional anatomy of the 12 pairs of **cranial nerves**. Because they will crop up again and again, it is a good plan to start with a really simple overview. First, learn the cranial nerves by name, number and by Roman numeral. Then learn about their functions: some are mixed (e.g. CN V), some entirely sensory (CN II), some entirely motor (e.g. CN VI), and some carry hitchhiking parasympathetic fibres (e.g. CN VII). Build on this foundation when a particular nerve is mentioned and make a final review of the nerves and their courses when you finish. This leads to some of the most detailed anatomy you will study; however, this knowledge is *needed* for neurological examinations.

If a nerve seems vulnerable in position it is possible to anticipate what problems might arise. For example, the course of the facial nerve (CN VII) lies first in a bony canal in the petrous temporal bone, where it gives off branches to the taste buds of the tongue and to the lacrimal gland. When it emerges from the skull, it is embedded in the parotid gland and is an entirely motor nerve to the muscles of facial expression. If it is compressed in the facial canal, then all its functions will be affected, leading to loss of taste, tear formation and paralysis of facial muscles; if, however, it is affected by disease of the parotid gland, then only the motor function will be lost while taste and tear formation are unaffected.

The innervation, blood supply and venous drainage of the face, scalp and orbit are regions that follow logically from an initial review of the cranial nerves. The common carotid artery has no branches. It divides at the level of C3 to form the external carotid artery, which supplies the face, neck, scalp and skull bones and the internal carotid, which supplies the brain together with the vertebral arteries. The vertebral arteries enter the cranium through the foramen magnum and supply the posterior parts of the brain before anastomosing with the internal carotid arteries at the **circle of Willis** (p. 139). The formation and arrangement of the **dural venous sinuses**, which drain the cranium, are quite difficult to visualize in three dimensions but are very important in understanding head injury.

Illustrations of the neck can be bewildering in their complexity. A good study plan is to look at a cross-section at C6 and think of it as five columns defined by tubes of fascia (p. 154). The supporting *bony muscular column* lies posteriorly; anterior to that is the **visceral column**, with the trachea, oesophagus and associated structures. On either side are the carotid sheaths with the common carotid arteries, internal jugular veins and vagus nerves. The fifth column is the entire neck wrapped around by investing fascia.

Table 1.2 THE PATHWAYS IN THE PHARYNX

Airway	Food passage	Feature
Nasal cavity	Oral cavity	Separated by hard palate
Nasopharynx	Oral cavity	Separated by soft palate
Oropharynx	Oropharynx	Common to airway and digestive systems
Laryngopharynx	Laryngopharynx	Common to airway and digestive systems
Larynx Trachea	Oesophagus	Cross-over point

The *cervical region* of the vertebral column is so mobile that there is considerable wear and tear on the facet joints. This can cause debilitating neck pain and may also affect the upper limb because the ventral rami of C_5, C_6, C_7, C_8 all contribute to the brachial plexus.

The major components of the visceral column of the neck are the midline structures that make up the airway and the food passages; they both begin in the facial part of the skull. *In order to perform effective airway management and life-support procedures, it is absolutely essential to understand that these vital pathways cross in the pharynx* (Table 1.2).

■ THE NERVOUS SYSTEM

What you need to know about nerves

Begin a study of the nervous system by learning its major functional divisions (Fig. 1.2).

It is important to understand what *structures* a nerve supplies (known as its **distribution**) and the *route* it takes to its destination (known as its **course**). The sites where a nerve is vulnerable to damage are obviously important (e.g. where a nerve is in direct contact with a bone and where a clinical procedure such as venepuncture is performed).

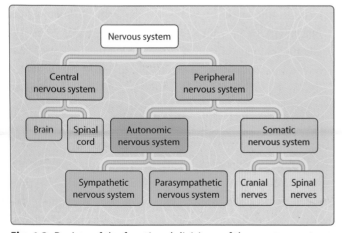

Fig. 1.2 Review of the functional divisions of the nervous system.

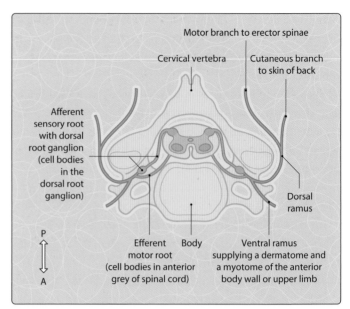

Fig. 1.3 Transverse section through the cervical spine showing the spinal cord and the formation of a pair of spinal nerves.

Each spinal nerve arises from two **roots**, the ventral (anterior) root carries motor fibres and the dorsal (posterior) root receives sensory fibres. The roots unite to form a *mixed* spinal nerve (i.e. both motor and sensory) as it emerges from the intervertebral foramen. Each spinal nerve then quickly divides to form a **dorsal ramus**, which supplies the dorsal body wall, and a **ventral ramus**, which supplies the ventral body wall and the limbs (Fig. 1.3). This arrangement is referred to and is relevant over and over again; learn it early.

Segmentation and the distribution of peripheral nerves

Early development of the nervous system involves the formation of the brain and neural tube with pairs of **somites** organizing externally along the body axis. It may not be immediately obvious but some systems retain features of this embryonic segmentation.

The brain, head and main sense organs are highly specialized and although an embryological background can provide a basis for understanding, the organization of these structures remains complicated. However, knowing that a somite consists of a block of muscle tissue with its own nerve and blood supply should help in understanding the distribution of peripheral nerves and blood vessels in the body wall.

The clearest example of segmental organization postnatally is the structure of the vertebral column, consisting of 33 individual bones each associated with a spinal nerve. In this book, each bone is referred to by its locations (T for thoracic, etc.) and a number (e.g. T3). The formation of spinal nerves reflects the functional segments of the spinal cord; spinal segments are named in relation to the adjacent vertebrae (nerves are given subscript numbers for clarity, e.g. T_3). The body wall, therefore, receives its nerve supply in a linear sequence, but because the limbs are outgrowths of the body wall, their organization seems less obvious; however, understanding the early pattern does explain the dermatome patterns and the distribution of peripheral nerves, which is the basis of neurological examination of patients.

Dermatomes and myotomes

In the cervical region, the nerves are named according to the vertebra *below* but from the first thoracic vertebra the nerves are named according to the vertebra *above*. This leads to the odd situation of having seven cervical vertebrae but eight cervical nerves (Fig. 1.4). It also means that in the thoracic region spinal (intercostal) nerves run *below* their own numbered rib.

In the thoracic region, it is easy to appreciate that each segmental nerve supplies the structures between the ribs; the motor fibres supply the strips of muscle between the ribs (intercostal muscles) and the skin that overlies the muscles is supplied by the sensory fibres. A group of muscles supplied by a single spinal nerve is known as a **myotome** and a strip of skin supplied by a single spinal segment is a **dermatome** (Figs 1.5–1.8). Knowledge of myotomes and dermatomes is very useful when there may have been damage to the spinal nerves (rather than peripheral nerves) or to the cord itself (e.g. after disc prolapse or spinal injury).

The dermatomes of the trunk are arranged in linear sequence; however, notice that at the sternal angle C_4 lies next to T_2; this is because the intervening segments are distributed over the upper limbs (Fig. 1.5). On the upper limb, the dermatomes are arranged around a central axis, with C_7 supplying the middle finger (Figs 1.5 and 1.7). The pattern appears more complicated in the lower limb because the lower limbs undergo medial rotation during development (Figs 1.5 and 1.7).

With a basic knowledge of the linear sequence, the dermatomes can be deduced from three reference points:

- C_7: middle finger
- T_{10}: umbilicus
- L_5: big toe.

Nerve plexuses

The segmental pattern of nerve distribution seen in the trunk is modified in the limbs. The ventral rami of spinal nerves combine

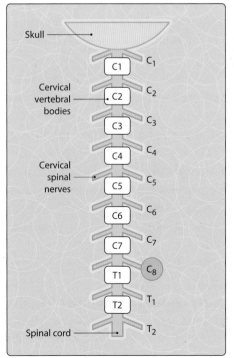

Fig. 1.4 Relationship of cervical, upper thoracic nerves and vertebrae.

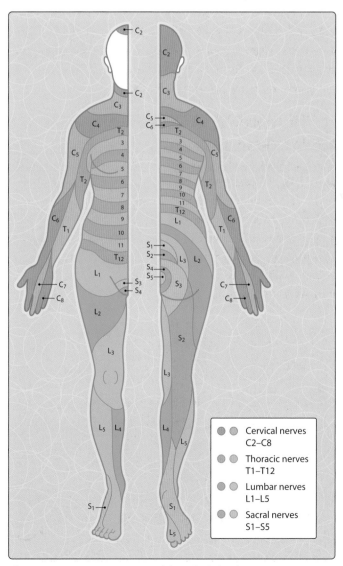

Fig. 1.5 Dermatome pattern of the whole body: anterior view (left) and posterior view (right).

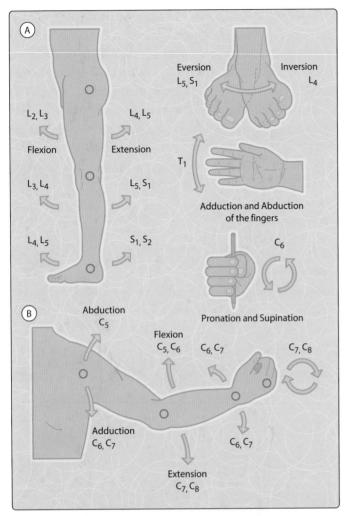

Fig. 1.6 Myotomes of the limbs. (A) Lower limb; (B) upper limb.

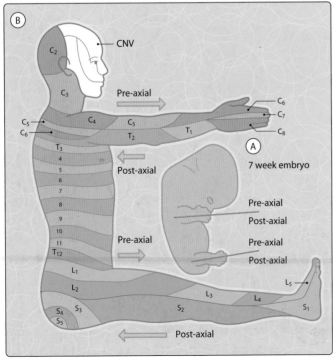

Fig. 1.7 The linear arrangement of dermatomes around the axial lines of the limbs. (A) 7-week embryo; (B) adult.

to form larger **trunks**, which then separate into **anterior divisions**, which supply flexor muscles, and **posterior divisions**, which supply extensor muscles. Generally, flexor muscles have a richer nerve supply and the skin over them is more sensitive and less hairy than that of extensor muscles (examine your forearm and hand). The final division into **terminal branches** ensures *motor* nerves are distributed so that:

- muscles in a compartment of the limb are all supplied by the same nerve (flexors of the arm are supplied by the musculo-cutaneous nerve)
- the nerve usually comprises fibres from two adjacent spinal segments (the musculocutaneous nerve carries C_5 and C_6)
- each spinal segment contributes to more than one named nerve (C_5 fibres are carried in musculocutaneous, axillary, suprascapular, subscapular, thoracodorsal, radial and median nerves (p. 40).

In the same way, *cutaneous* (i.e. sensory) nerves also receive fibres from more than one spinal segment (e.g. the lateral cutaneous nerve of the forearm carries fibres from both C_5 and C_6). This means that, in addition to being able to map out dermatomes on the body surface, it is also possible to make a map of the distribution of *named cutaneous nerves*. The two maps are not the same; this is a quite difficult concept and needs some thought.

Autonomic nerves

The autonomic system (Fig. 1.2) controls all those processes over which we have no voluntary control (rate of heart beat, digestion, temperature control, etc.). The system consists of sympathetic and parasympathetic nerves, which sometimes act antagonistically; for example, sympathetic stimulation raises the heart rate whereas parasympathetic stimulation lowers it. The details of autonomic nerves are important but difficult. Two general principles will help.

1. Sympathetic stimulation elicits the 'fight or flight' response; it brings about the consumption of energy and controls body temperature through structures in the skin (blood vessels, sweat glands). Sympathetic fibres are distributed in *every spinal nerve* in order to reach these skin structures (p. 74).
2. Parasympathetic stimulation promotes 'rest and digest'. It brings about conservation of energy and supplies the viscera. Parasympathetic fibres are distributed via four cranial (III, VII, IX and X) and three sacral nerves $S_2–S_4$ only; they *do not* supply the limbs (see p. 72).

Cranial nerves

The 12 cranial nerves are numbered in the order they arise from the brainstem (Fig. 1.8). Table 3.56.1 (p. 136) gives more details of each nerve.

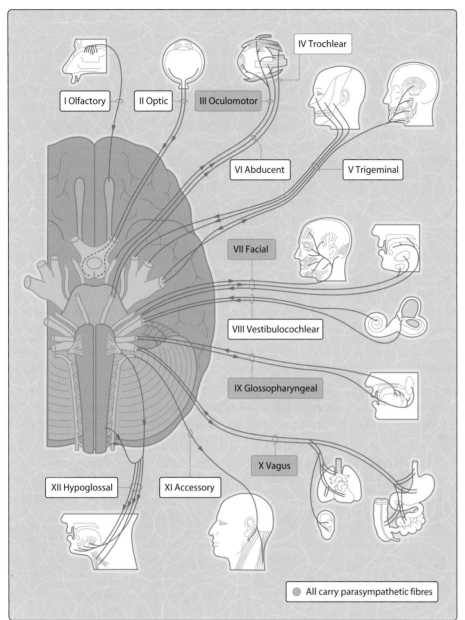

Fig. 1.8 Pictorial representation of the cranial nerves.

Labels in figure:
- I Olfactory
- II Optic
- III Oculomotor
- IV Trochlear
- VI Abducent
- V Trigeminal
- VII Facial
- VIII Vestibulocochlear
- IX Glossopharyngeal
- X Vagus
- XII Hypoglossal
- XI Accessory
- All carry parasympathetic fibres

■ THE CARDIOVASCULAR SYSTEM AND LYMPH VESSELS

What you need to know about the heart and blood vessels

The heart functions as two pumps that deliver the same volume of blood but at different pressures. The right side of the heart receives deoxygenated blood from the body and pumps it to the lungs at approximately 35 mmHg. It is oxygenated in the lungs and returned to the left side of the heart (**pulmonary circulation**). The left heart pumps blood to all the systems of the body at approximately 120 mmHg (**systemic circulation**). Examination of the heart is an essential component of clinical examination and *you must learn the surface markings of the borders and valves.*

Arteries generally carry blood away from the heart, and their pulsations can be felt through their walls. *You should learn the major arteries, where they begin and end, their course, distribution and pulse points.* Around the joints, arteries are interconnected by branches (**anastomoses**) that allow the blood to bypass the major route if it is obstructed in some way (developing a **collateral circulation**). Some arteries have either no interconnections (e.g. arcuate arteries of the kidney, central artery of the retina) or poor anastomoses (e.g. coronary arteries). They are **end arteries** and a blockage will result in tissue damage (infarction).

Veins are more variable than arteries and have thinner walls. Superficial veins lie in superficial fascia and are often visible through the skin; clinically they are used for venepuncture and insertion of catheters. Important sites for venepuncture are:

- dorsal venous arch of the hand
- cephalic
- median cubital
- great saphenous
- femoral
- internal jugular
- subclavian
- brachiocephalic.

Deep veins (venae comitantes) lie alongside arteries within the fascial compartments in the limbs; they are particularly important in the lower limb (p. 109). Venous blood from the gut is rich in nutrients and drains to the liver via the hepatic portal vein. The products of digestion are metabolized by the liver and the blood is returned to the heart in the inferior vena cava (**portal system**).

Lymphatic drainage of the body as a whole

Knowledge of lymphatic drainage of the body is of great clinical importance. Disease, including cancer, can spread along lymphatic vessels from one organ to another or to distant lymph nodes. It is important to learn the main lymphatics of the body and the position of lymph nodes. It is also important to know the route taken by lymph draining from any particular region or viscus and through which nodes it passes (Fig. 1.9).

At the arterial end of blood capillaries, the hydrostatic blood pressure forces water and electrolytes out of the capillaries into the extracellular spaces. At the venous end, fluid tends to be drawn back into the venules; however, there is usually more tissue fluid formed than returns at the venous end. The excess fluid is **lymph** and this drains into a series of **lymphatic capillaries**, which form a vast network of vessels throughout the body *except* in the central nervous system, bone, bone marrow, cartilage, cornea, teeth and placenta. Lymph is a clear fluid that contains cells, cellular debris and cell products such as hormones; it may contain pathogens. In the gut, lymphatic capillaries or **lacteals** form the core of intestinal villi. The lymph from the gut is known as **chyle**; it is milky because it contains emulsified products of fat digestion.

Thin-walled lymphatics converge to form progressively larger diameter trunks with numerous valves to prevent back flow. Superficial lymphatics accompany veins while deep lymph vessels are associated with arteries. The movement of lymph comes from the squeezing action of adjacent muscles and arteries. Eventually all the lymph is returned to the venous circulation in the neck.

Along the course of lymphatics are aggregations of lymphoid tissue, which form groups of **lymph nodes**. Lymphocytes in the nodes sample the fluid for antigens and can initiate an immune response. Resting nodes are just a few millimetres in length, but when they are activated they can increase greatly in size. Some nodes are deep within the trunk (e.g. para-aortic); others are superficial and may be palpable (e.g. inguinal, axillary and cervical nodes; Fig. 1.9).

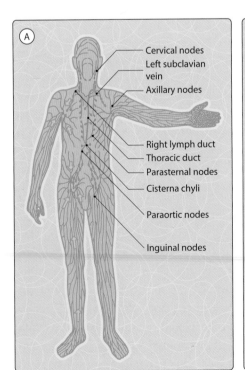

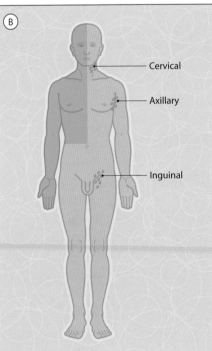

Fig. 1.9 Lymphatics and lymph nodes of the body. (A) General plan of the lymphatic system (arrows show the direction of superficial drainage); (B) palpable lymphatic nodes (shaded area of the body is drained by the right lymphatic duct).

Lymph drainage converges on two pathways.

1. Lymph from the right upper limb and the right side of the head, neck and upper thorax drains to the right lymph duct, which enters the venous system at the junction of the right internal jugular and right subclavian veins.

2. Lymph from the lower part of the body drains to the **cisterna chyli** (a reservoir that lies on the lumbar vertebrae just inferior to the diaphragm) and then to the **thoracic duct**, which eventually empties into the junction of the left internal jugular and left subclavian veins in the neck (p. 141). Lymph from the left upper limb and the left side of the head and neck drains into the thoracic duct, from which it empties into the venous system.

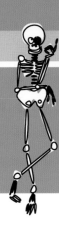

High return facts

General principles

1 Anatomical terms are the basis of the professional language used in written medical reports and when talking with colleagues. They are specific and unambiguous; you cannot escape knowing them! Learn them at an early stage; do not be afraid to use them whenever you can, even if you are unsure how to pronounce them!

2 The vertebral column protects the spinal cord, provides support for the skull and confers flexibility through the articulation of 33 individual vertebrae. Each of its five regions has different modifications relating to different functional constraints (e.g. each thoracic vertebra articulates with a pair of ribs). The column is supported by a series of longitudinal ligaments. Between each vertebral body is an intervertebral disc consisting of a central nucleus pulposus and an outer annulus fibrosus. The structure of the disc and its close relations are important in understanding the effects of a prolapsed (slipped) disc. For example, the intervertebral disc is prone to age-related degenerative change that weakens the annulus and allows the nucleus to prolapse and press on the adjacent spinal nerve.

3 The central nervous system consists of the brain and spinal cord. The cranial nerves and spinal nerves make up the peripheral nervous system. The spinal nerves reflect the early arrangement of segments in the embryo. Each segment of the spinal cord gives rise to dorsal (sensory) and ventral (motor) roots that unite within the vertebral canal to form a pair of spinal nerves. As they emerge from their intervertebral foramen, the spinal nerves divide into dorsal and ventral rami. The dorsal rami supply the skin and muscles of the back. The ventral rami supply the anterior body wall and undergo specific and complex branching to form the plexuses that supply the limbs. Knowledge of the distribution of spinal nerves to the skin (dermatomes) and to muscles (myotomes) is important when there is suspected damage to the spinal cord or spinal nerves. The spinal cord and brain are surrounded by the meninges. In adults, the spinal cord only reaches as far as L1/L2; the remainder of the vertebral canal is occupied by the spinal roots of lumbar and sacral nerves. Lumbar puncture is performed at the level of L3/L4.

Upper limb

4 The bones and joints of the upper limb are commonly damaged as the arms are used for protection in a fall or during traumatic injury. The limb has only one small bony joint with the sternum and is mainly attached by muscles. This arrangement allows extraordinary mobility—but at the cost of stability.

5 The axilla is a pyramidal space between the thorax wall and the proximal part of the humerus. It is the gateway between the limb and the neck through which neurovascular structures pass. Powerful muscles form the anterior and posterior walls of the axilla. Movements of the scapula on the thorax wall greatly increase the range of abduction.

6 The subclavian artery is the only arterial supply to the upper limb. However, since there are rich anastomoses in the scapula region, around the elbow and in the hand, trauma rarely results in ischaemia. The positions of the pulses are important in clinical examination including the measurement of blood pressure.

7 It is important to know the position of superficial veins that are commonly used for venepuncture. Lymph from the upper limb and thorax wall drains to the axillary nodes, which drain via the apical nodes to the thoracic duct on the left and to the right lymph duct. Both ducts drain into the venous system at the junction of the internal jugular and subclavian veins. Three-quarters of the lymph from the breast drains to the axillary nodes, which, therefore, are a common site for the metastatic spread of breast cancer.

8 The nerve supply to the skin and muscles of the upper limb is from branches of the brachial plexus. The plexus comprises the ventral rami of cervical spinal nerves C_5–T_1. The proximal muscles are supplied by the upper roots of the brachial plexus (e.g. the muscles acting on the shoulder are supplied by C_5 and C_6). The distal muscles are supplied by the lower roots of the brachial plexus (e.g. the intrinsic muscles of the hand are supplied by T_1). There are five terminal branches: the musculocutaneous, median, ulnar, axillary and radial nerves. The trunks of the brachial plexus lie in the posterior triangle of the neck and can be damaged in traction injuries.

9 The glenohumeral joint has the greatest range of movement of any joint in the body and is the most commonly dislocated. Three factors enhance its mobility and contribute to its instability: limited bony contact (only one-third of the humeral head is in contact with the glenoid fossa), ligamentous support (the capsule is loose, ligaments only providing support superiorly and anteriorly) and muscular support (rotator cuff muscles hold the head of the humerus in the glenoid cavity). The joint is weakest inferiorly and is most vulnerable in the abducted position. Dislocation may cause damage to the axillary nerve, leading to paralysis of deltoid and loss of sensation over deltoid.

10 The arm is divided by fascial septa into an anterior (flexor) compartment supplied by the musculocutaneous nerve and a posterior (extensor) compartment supplied by the radial nerve. The axillary, radial and ulnar nerves lie in direct contact with the humerus and are vulnerable to damage in fractures. The median nerve, brachial artery and tendon of biceps lie in the cubital fossa. The median cubital vein is superficial and a common site for venepuncture. Blood pressure measurements are made over the brachial artery. The elbow is a stable joint between the humerus, radius and ulna, all three bones articulating within one joint capsule.

11 The forearm is divided into flexor and extensor compartments. The flexor compartment contains the long flexor muscles; they are all supplied by the median nerve *except* flexor carpi ulnaris and the medial half of flexor digitorum profundus (supplied by the ulnar nerve). The extensor compartment is organized in the same way as the flexor compartment and is supplied by the terminal branch of the radial nerve (posterior interosseous nerve). If the radial nerve is damaged, it may impair wrist and finger extension causing wrist drop. The anatomical snuff box is a hollow at the base of the thumb between the long tendons of the thumb where the scaphoid and radial styloid can be palpated.

12 The carpal tunnel is formed by the attachment of flexor retinaculum to the scaphoid and trapezium laterally and the pisiform and hamate medially. It contains nine tendons and the median nerve. Compression of the median nerve in the tunnel leads to carpal tunnel syndrome (tingling in the lateral $3\frac{1}{2}$ digits, with weakness and wasting of the thenar muscles). Because the wrist and hand are so commonly damaged, it is important to understand the organization of the neurovascular structures both at the wrist and within the palm. The arteries and nerves are superficial and commonly damaged.

13 Movements of the digits are complex and depend on the long flexors and the small muscles that arise within the hand. All of the small muscles are supplied by the ulnar nerve *except* the thenar muscles, which are supplied by the median nerve (both carry fibres from the T_1 spinal segment). The median nerve also gives a sensory supply to the lateral side of the palm, the palmar surface of the lateral $3\frac{1}{2}$ digits and their nail beds, while the ulnar nerve supplies the medial side of the palm and the medial $1\frac{1}{2}$ digits and their nail beds. On the dorsum of the hand, the skin over the lateral $3\frac{1}{2}$ digits is supplied by the radial nerve and the skin over the medial $1\frac{1}{2}$ digits is supplied by the ulnar nerve. The interossei and lumbrical muscles acting together flex the metacarpophalangeal joints and extend the interphalangeal joints. If the intrinsic muscles are paralysed, the unapposed long flexors and extensors cause hyperextension of the metacarpophalangeal joints and flexion of the interphalangeal joints (claw hand).

14 Problems relating to specific nerve roots C_5–T_1 will give rise to particular clinical signs in the upper limbs. Clinical testing of these nerve roots involves examination of myotomes, dermatomes and tendon reflexes of the upper limb. Because the motor supply to the diaphragm is mainly from C_4, lying immediately above the roots controlling the upper limb, testing of the upper limb will help in the assessment of a neck injury that could interfere with breathing.

Thorax

15 You need a good knowledge of the thoracic cage to be able to relate bony landmarks to the position of thoracic viscera when you examine the thorax or interpret radiographs, magnetic resonance imaging or computed tomography of the chest. The thoracic cage consists of 12 pairs of ribs that articulate posteriorly with the bodies and transverse processes of the 12 thoracic vertebrae. Anteriorly, the costal cartilages of the first seven ribs articulate directly with the sternum, ribs 8–10 are shorter and their costal cartilages articulate with the one above to form the costal margin. Ribs 11 and 12 are so short that they do not articulate anteriorly. The joints between the ribs and the vertebrae allow breathing movements. The rib cage overlaps abdominal viscera such as the kidneys and liver.

16 The early segmental arrangement of the body wall persists in the thorax. The intercostal space is filled by three layers of intercostal muscles, which lift the rib below towards the rib above. Each space receives a segmental nerve supply from an intercostal nerve carrying motor fibres to the intercostal muscles and sensory fibres from the adjacent skin and parietal pleura. The spaces also receive a segmental blood supply from the aorta posteriorly and anteriorly from the internal thoracic artery, a branch of the subclavian, which continues inferiorly to supply the anterior abdominal wall. Venous drainage posteriorly is via the azygos system; anteriorly it mirrors the arterial supply. The neurovascular bundle lies in the superior part of the intercostal space, under the rib between the middle and inner layers of muscle.

17 Contraction of the intercostal muscles and diaphragm causes movements that increase the volume of the thorax, lower the internal pressure and draw air into the lungs. Expiration is usually a passive process that depends on elastic recoil of the lungs and airways. The pleural cavities on either side of the mediastinum are lined by parietal pleura, which adheres to the inner surface of the thorax wall, and visceral pleura, which covers all the surfaces of the lungs. Slight negative pressure between the membranes maintains surface tension between the membranes and ensures that the lungs inflate as the chest wall moves during inspiration. The surface markings of the pleural cavities are important, particularly because they extend above the clavicles into the root of the neck and below the rib cage (costomediastinal recesses).

18 Air is drawn into the lungs along the branches of the airway known as the bronchial tree. The trachea divides into two main bronchi at the level of the sternal angle, the right main bronchus divides into three lobar bronchi (one to each of three lobes) and the left into two (one to each of two lobes). The lobar bronchi divide again into segmental bronchi (10 on the right and nine on the left), which supply functionally separate segments. The final branching (bronchioles and alveoli) of the airway brings the inspired air in the alveoli into very close contact with pulmonary capillaries and facilitates gaseous exchange. Lymphatic drainage of the lungs is important because of the high incidence of lung cancer.

19 The middle mediastinum lies behind the body of the sternum and consists of the contents of the pericardium. The fibrous pericardium is attached superiorly to the great vessels and inferiorly to the diaphragm. The parietal and visceral layers of the serous pericardium line the inner aspect of the fibrous layer and the surface of the heart. The right and left sides of the heart are completely separated from each other. The right side pumps to the pulmonary circulation and the left to the systemic circulation. Each side is divided into two chambers by an atrioventricular valve, which ensures one-way flow of blood through the heart. Knowledge of the surface markings of the heart and an understanding of which chambers appear on which borders is essential for the interpretation of a chest radiograph.

20 The myocardium receives a rich blood supply to support its constant activity. The right and left coronary arteries arise from the ascending aorta just above the aortic valve. They lie, embedded in fat, in the grooves between the chambers of the heart. The two arteries are connected by anastomoses; however, the calibre of the anastomosing vessels is very narrow and sudden occlusion may result in myocardial infarction. Their pattern of distribution is important, particularly in relation to the conducting system that carries the cardiac impulse from the sinuatrial node to the myocardium.

21 The superior mediastinum lies above the plane between the sternal angle and T4. It is a complex region linking thoracic anatomy at the root of the neck with the upper limbs. The key to this region is to realize that the structures that lie on the first rib reflect the relations of the great vessels in the superior mediastinum (subclavian vein is the most anterior structure with the subclavian artery behind it and posteriorly is the inferior trunk of the brachial plexus). The venous plane lies anterior to the arterial plane and the phrenic and vagus nerves, passing from the neck to the thorax, lie between them. Asymmetry of thoracic vascular structures relates to the fact that, in general, *veins* return blood to the right heart and *arteries* leave the left heart. Thus the right phrenic nerve will be related to veins (inferior and superior vena cavae) while the left phrenic nerve is related to arteries (left common carotid, left subclavian and aorta).

22 The structures that lie in the posterior mediastinum lie anterior to the vertebral bodies of T5–T12. The oesophagus begins in the neck (C_6), where it lies posterior to the trachea and passes behind the left principal bronchus and left atrium before passing through the muscular part of the left hemidiaphragm at the level of T10 with the vagal trunks and left gastric vessels. The aorta, thoracic duct, azygos and hemiazygos veins pass behind the diaphragm at the level of T12.

23 The diaphragm separates the thorax from the abdomen and is pierced by the structures that pass between these two regions. The fibrous pericardium is attached to the central tendon, which is pierced by the inferior vena cava and right phrenic nerve (T8). The oesophagus and left gastric vessels pierce the muscular part of the left side of the diaphragm (T10). The *right* crus forms a sling around the inferior part of the oesophagus that helps to prevent gastric reflux. The aorta, thoracic duct, azygos and hemiazygos veins pass behind the diaphragm at the level of T12. The phrenic nerves (C_3, C_4, C_5 'keep the diaphragm alive') are the *only* motor supply to the diaphragm and also give a sensory supply to the central tendon, pericardium, pleura and diaphragmatic peritoneum.

24 The functions of the body that are not under voluntary control are innervated by the autonomic nervous system. It has two divisions that often act antagonistically: sympathetic nerves tending to speed things up and parasympathetic nerves tending to slow things down. Activation of the latter conserves energy by promoting 'rest and digest'. Parasympathetic neurones lie either in the brainstem nuclei of cranial nerves III, VII, IX and X or in the sacral region of the spinal cord S_2, S_3, S_4. The vagus nerve (CN X) emerges from the skull, passes inferiorly through the neck and enters the thorax, giving important branches to the heart, lungs oesophagus and the intrinsic muscles of the larynx (recurrent laryngeal nerves). It carries preganglionic parasympathetic fibres and the neurones synapse in ganglia close to the organ they supply.

25 Activation of the sympathetic system consumes energy and prepares the body for 'fight or flight'. Sympathetic nerve fibres must 'hitch hike' with *every* spinal nerve in order to reach their destinations, such as structures in the skin. Sympathetic neurones lie in the lateral grey of the spinal cord between T1 and L2, pass from the cord in the ventral root of a spinal nerve and enter a ganglion of the sympathetic trunk via a white ramus communicans. They synapse and pass into spinal nerves via a grey ramus communicans to supply the body wall. Unnamed visceral branches also arise from the sympathetic trunk to supply thoracic viscera; abdominal viscera are supplied by branches known as splanchnic nerves.

Abdomen and pelvis

26 The anatomy of the abdominal wall is important because it is frequently examined and is the basis for surgical incisions. The wall consists of three layers of muscle (external and internal oblique and transversus abdominis). Their muscle fibres give way anteriorly to tendinous sheets that enclose the rectus abdominis muscle (rectus sheath). They meet in the midline at the linea alba. The anterior abdominal wall is supplied by intercostal nerves T_7–T_{12} and L_1. The nerves branch and are interconnected so their motor and sensory distributions overlap. The abdominal wall receives a segmental supply posteriorly from the intercostal branches of the aorta and anteriorly from the superior and inferior epigastric arteries, which lie within the rectus sheath.

27 During fetal development, the gonads lie in the abdomen close to the primitive kidney. In the inferior part of the abdomen, a finger-like process of the peritoneum (processus vaginalis) pushes out through the abdominal wall, extending the three layers of the wall in front of it and forming the basic structure of the inguinal canal. In males just before birth, the testis migrates through the canal into the scrotum, dragging behind it the spermatic cord containing the testicular artery, veins and lymphatics (NB testicular tumours *do not* metastasize to the inguinal nodes). The round ligament is the female equivalent but is much smaller. The inguinal canal is important because it is a weakness in the abdominal wall and inguinal hernias may develop in older men either as a congenital problem or later in life as the result of degenerative changes.

28 Parietal peritoneum is the serous membrane that lines the abdominal cavity; where it is reflected off the wall onto the abdominal organs it becomes the visceral layer. Some organs are 'plastered down' onto the posterior abdominal wall by the peritoneum and are referred to as retroperitoneal (e.g. kidney). Others are suspended in folds of peritoneum (mesenteries). Mesentery, omentum, ligament and epiploic all mean the same thing: a double layer of visceral peritoneum that connects a viscus to the body wall and carries blood vessels, lymphatics and nodes, nerves and fat. Some viscera have two mesenteries (stomach, liver, spleen and colon); others have only one (small intestine). The space between the parietal and visceral peritoneum is the peritoneal cavity, which is kidney shaped with deep paravertebral gutters on either side. It is divided into the lesser sac (behind the stomach) and greater sac (greater part of the cavity). For the purposes of description, the cavity is also described as being divided by the transverse mesocolon into the supra- and infracolic compartments.

29 The coeliac trunk supplies the foregut (i.e. inferior one-third of the oesophagus, stomach and duodenum as far as the major duodenal papilla (second part)). It also supplies the liver, spleen and most of the pancreas because they are foregut derivatives. The superior mesenteric artery supplies the midgut (i.e. the rest of the pancreas, the inferior and ascending parts of the duodenum, jejunum, ilium, caecum, appendix, ascending colon and the proximal two-thirds of the transverse colon). The inferior mesenteric artery supplies the hindgut (i.e. distal one-third of the transverse colon, descending and sigmoid colon, rectum and as far as the upper part of the anal canal).

30 The portal vein and its tributaries carry one-third of the body's total blood volume. It drains all of the intestines (except the lowest part of the rectum and anal canal), spleen, pancreas and gall bladder. It is unusual because the blood that it carries originates from the intestinal capillary bed, where it has picked up the products of digestion, and will pass through a *second* capillary bed in the liver before returning to the heart. There are three important regions where there are connections between portal and systemic veins

- gastro-oesophageal junction
- paraumbilical region
- rectum and anal canal.

31 The stomach is relatively fixed: at the cardia by the passage of the oesophagus through the diaphragm and at the pylorus because here the duodenum becomes retroperitoneal. Because the body of the stomach is suspended by two mesenteries, its shape and position varies between individuals. The lesser omentum, which runs from the lesser curvature to the liver, contains the left and right gastric vessels and the greater omentum, which lies between the stomach, transverse colon and the posterior abdominal wall, contains the right and left gastroepiploic arteries. Internally, the lining of the stomach is arranged in folds (rugae), which allow considerable expansion to accommodate ingested food and gastric secretions. The duodenum is retroperitoneal and C shaped, curving around the head of the pancreas. The common bile duct and pancreatic duct open together into its second part, which marks the boundary between the embryonic foregut and midgut. The fourth part becomes the jejunum at the duodenojejunal flexure.

32 The liver lies in the right hypochondrium and epigastric regions and is overlapped by the right costal margin. Its diaphragmatic surface abuts the right hemidiaphragm. Inferiorly, the visceral surface is covered by peritoneum and there are important peritoneal recesses between the liver, diaphragm and kidney. The porta hepatis is the point of entry of the hepatic artery (carrying oxygenated blood) and the hepatic portal vein (carrying the venous blood from the intestines) and also where the hepatic ducts (carrying bile) leave the liver. The hepatic ducts join together to form the common hepatic duct, which carries bile to the gall bladder. The gall bladder lies on the undersurface of the liver behind the tip of the ninth right costal cartilage. Bile is released into the second part of the duodenum via the common bile duct. The common bile duct lies with the hepatic artery and hepatic portal vein in the free edge of the lesser omentum that forms the anterior border of the opening of the epiploic foramen. The common bile duct joins the pancreatic duct and they empty together at the major duodenal papilla.

33 The head of the pancreas lies in the curve of the duodenum and its duct opens with the common bile duct into the second part of the duodenum at the major duodenal papilla. The body lies in the transpyloric plane and its tail extends in the lienorenal ligament as far as the hilum of the spleen. The superior mesenteric vessels first lie behind and then hook anteriorly over the uncinate process. The splenic and inferior mesenteric veins join behind the neck of the pancreas to form the hepatic portal vein. The stomach and lesser sac lie anterior to the pancreas; the inferior vena cava, aorta, coeliac plexus, left kidney and suprarenal gland (with their vessels) all lie posteriorly. The splenic artery passes to the left across the superior border of the pancreas to the hilum of the spleen. The spleen lies under the left dome of the diaphragm with its long axis lying along the 10th rib. It is separated from the ribs by the diaphragm and costodiaphragmatic pleural recess. The spleen is not normally palpable.

34 An understanding of the embryonic rotation of the gut is helpful in understanding the postnatal arrangement of the gut tube and its blood supply. The midgut comprises the jejunum, ilium, caecum, ascending colon and two-thirds of the transverse colon. The jejunum and ilium are suspended by mesentery, which has a short proximal origin from the posterior abdominal wall but fans out distally to support 6 m of intestine supplied by branches of the superior mesenteric artery. The ascending and descending limbs of the colon are retroperitoneal while the transverse colon is mobile and suspended from the transverse mesocolon. The appendix is variable in position but normally located behind the caecum. The hindgut comprises the remainder of the transverse colon, descending colon, sigmoid colon, rectum and first part of the anal canal. It is supplied by branches of the inferior mesenteric artery.

35 The kidneys develop in the pelvis and migrate upwards during development. They lie in contact with the diaphragm and are overlapped by the 12th ribs. The right kidney lies behind the liver, duodenum and ascending colon; the left lies behind the stomach, spleen, pancreas, jejunum and descending colon. The renal arteries are large direct branches that enter the hilum of the kidneys in the transpyloric plane and the terminal branches are end arteries. The ureters lie retroperitoneally. They begin at the renal pelvis, cross the pelvic brim at the sacroiliac joint and end by piercing the bladder wall obliquely at the superior angles of the trigone. The development of the adrenals is complex and they receive blood from three arteries.

36 The posterior abdominal wall is supported by the lumbar spine and sacrum. The prevertebral (flexor) muscles, quadratus lumborum, iliacus and psoas major and minor, receive segmental nerves and arteries. The lumbar plexus gives branches that supply the lower part of the anterior abdominal wall and the femoral and obturator nerves, which supply the lower limb, and contributes to the sacral plexus. The abdominal viscera receive an autonomic supply from the sympathetic and parasympathetic nervous systems. The autonomic plexuses are associated with the anterior branches of the aorta (coeliac, superior mesenteric and inferior mesenteric arteries). The sympathetic supply arises from the greater, lesser and least splanchnic nerves, which arise in the thorax and synapse in the abdominal plexuses. The parasympathetic supply is from the vagus nerves as far as the splenic flexure and more distally arise from pelvic splanchnic nerves (S_2–S_4).

37 The pelvic inlet is formed by the sacral promontory behind, the arcuate lines of the ilium and the pubic symphysis. The outlet is bounded by the coccyx, sacrotuberous ligaments, ischial tuberosities and pubic arch. The female pelvis is larger in all dimensions for obvious reasons. The levator ani and coccygeus muscles form the pelvic floor (or diaphragm), which divides the pelvic cavity from the perineum below. It is important because it supports pelvic viscera and forms part of the urinary and anal sphincters. The diaphragm is funnel shaped and the most inferior part (between the vagina and anus in females) is the perineal body. The peritoneum forms ligaments and recesses between the pelvic organs. The pelvic organs are supplied by branches of the internal iliac artery and drain to the equivalent veins.

38 The perineum is the diamond-shaped area between the thighs. All perineal structures are supplied by the pudendal nerve and the internal pudendal artery. It is divided into two triangles. The posterior or anal triangle is the same in both sexes and contains the anal canal with the ischioanal fossae on either side. The anatomy of the anal canal is important because it marks the boundary between the gut tube and the outside of the body. The ischioanal fossae are fat-filled spaces that contain the pudendal canals, which carry the pudendal nerve and internal pudendal artery. The anatomy of the urogenital triangle is complex but important. It is spanned by a sheet of voluntary muscle that surrounds the urethra and forms the external urinary sphincter. It also supports the vagina.

39 The ductus deferens lies within the spermatic cord. It transports sperm from the epididymis of the testis to the ampulla on the posterior surface of the bladder. It passes anteriorly, entering the prostate gland as the ejaculatory duct, which opens into the urethra at the base of the bladder. At ejaculation, sperm are suspended in seminal fluid released by the seminal vesicles and prostate glands. The prostate gland completely surrounds the prostatic urethra at the base of the bladder and is supported inferiorly by the levator ani. The membranous part of the urethra passes through the urogenital diaphragm and turning anteriorly is surrounded by the corpus spongiosum (spongy urethra). The penis consists of three columns of erectile tissue: two corpora cavernosae and the corpus

spongiosum, which is expanded distally to form the glans penis. The bladder lies below the level of the peritoneum and as it distends to store approximately 500 ml urine, it rises into the abdomen stripping the peritoneum from the anterior abdominal wall. The rectum and anal canal lie behind the bladder.

40 The ovaries develop in the upper part of the abdominal cavity and descend into the pelvic cavity, where they lie close to the obturator nerve on the lateral wall. Each month from puberty to menopause, an oocyte is released and is transported to the uterine cavity in the uterine tubes. The tubes and uterus are enclosed in the upper border of the broad ligament. The uterus is normally anteverted and anteflexed, lying above the superior surface of the bladder to form a narrow uterovesical pouch. Posteriorly, the rectouterine pouch is related to the posterior vaginal fornix. The cervix projects into the anterior wall of the vagina, where there is a squamocolumnar junction. Pregnancy and childbirth cause enormous strains on the uterus, cervix and vagina, which are supported by the pelvic diaphragm and fascial ligaments. The ureters pass forwards on either side of the cervix between the lateral vaginal fornices and uterine arteries. The bladder rests directly on the pelvic diaphragm. The external genitalia are homologous with the male structures. The much shorter urethra, which opens between the clitoris and vagina, predisposes women to ascending urinary tract infections.

Lower limb

41 The general plan of the lower limb is similar to the upper limb; however, during development the lower limb undergoes medial rotation, bringing the extensors anteriorly with the knee pointing forwards. The lower limb has a very firm attachment through the rigid pelvis to the vertebral column. The joints are relatively stable and influenced by the line of gravity; their major function is to transmit the forces generated by the powerful muscles of the lower limb.

42 The deep fascia of the lower limb is dense and inelastic; it forms a stocking around the muscles dividing them into compartments containing functional groups. Superficial veins are connected to deep veins within the compartments through a series of perforating veins with valves that ensure that blood flows from superficial to deep. Damage to the valves results in the development of varicose veins. The deep veins form a plexus within the soleus muscle of the calf. When soleus contracts, pressure in the compartment rises and blood is forced upwards, pulling blood from the superficial veins into the deep veins (calf muscle pump). The superficial inguinal lymph nodes drain the whole lower limb, external genitalia and perineum (with the important exception of the testes).

43 The lower limb is supplied by the femoral artery, which is a continuation of the external iliac artery, and by branches of the internal iliac artery, which supply the gluteal region. The femoral artery enters the thigh at the mid-inguinal point lying anterior to the hip joint. The powerful muscles of the thigh are largely supplied by the profunda femoris artery, while the main arterial stem passes under cover of the sartorius muscle, spiraling behind the knee to become the popliteal artery. The posterior tibial artery supplies the calf muscles and passes behind the medial malleolus to supply the foot. The anterior tibial artery supplies the anterior extensor compartment and terminates as the dorsalis pedis, which is palpable lateral to the extensor hallucis tendon.

44 The lower limb is supplied by the lumbar and sacral plexuses. The lumbar plexus consists of the ventral rami of spinal nerves L_1–L_4. Branches from the plexus supply flexors of the hip (iliacus, psoas) and the anterior abdominal wall. The femoral nerve supplies extensors of the knee and the skin of the anterior thigh, while the obturator nerve supplies adductors of the hip and skin of the medial thigh. The rest of the limb is supplied by branches of the sacral plexus L_4–S_4. The superior and inferior gluteal nerves supply the abductors and extensors of the hip. The posterior cutaneous nerve of thigh supplies skin over the buttock, perineum and posterior thigh. The sciatic nerve supplies the hamstrings and divides mid-thigh into the common fibular and tibial nerves. They supply the whole of the leg and foot except for the medial skin, which is supplied by the saphenous nerve (branch of the femoral nerve).

45 There are three compartments in the thigh. The extensors of the knee lie anteriorly and are supplied by the femoral nerve. The adductors are medial and are supplied by the obturator nerve; the flexors of the knee lie posteriorly and are supplied by the sciatic nerve. The femoral triangle lies inferior to the inguinal ligament on the anterior surface of the thigh. It contains superficial neurovascular structures: from lateral to medial they are the femoral nerve (lateral to femoral pulse), the femoral artery and the femoral vein medial to femoral pulse (remember NAVY: nerve, artery, vein, Y fronts!). The femoral canal is the most medial structure; it is a site of weakness in the anterior abdominal wall and is where a femoral hernia may develop below and lateral to the pubic tubercle.

46 A thick layer of superficial fascia covers the muscles of the gluteal region. Gluteus maximus is important in extending the hip from a flexed position (e.g. when you stand up from sitting or when walking up stairs). Gluteus medius and minimus maintain the horizontal position of the pelvis during walking. The region is the gateway to the posterior thigh for a number of important neurovascular structures that emerge from the pelvis through the greater sciatic foramen. The largest and most important structure is the sciatic nerve, which lies half way between posterior superior ischial spine and ischial tuberosity. Intermuscular injections are usually performed in the upper, lateral quadrant of the gluteal region to avoid damage to the sciatic nerve.

47 The hip joint is a stable ball and socket joint. Its stability results from the snug fit of the large femoral head and deep acetabulum, which is supported on all sides by powerful intrinsic ligaments and muscles. The joint carries the whole body weight and transmits the forces generated in locomotion. There is a tendency for the trunk to tilt backwards at the hip joints because the line of gravity passes posteriorly; this is resisted by the powerful iliofemoral ligament. In adults fractures of the narrow neck may damage the blood supply to the femoral head, resulting in avascular necrosis.

48 The knee is a modified hinge joint between the femur and tibia that allows some medial rotation in the fully extended position; it is commonly damaged in sporting activities. Like all hinge joints it has strong medial and lateral collateral ligaments to support the joint. In addition, it has important intra-articular ligaments. The posterior cruciate ligament prevents hyperflexion and supports the body weight when walking down stairs. The anterior cruciate ligament prevents hyperextension. Intra-articular cartilages are seen in joints that allow rotation (e.g. sternoclavicular). In the knee, the medial and lateral menisci act as cushions between the articular surfaces. The medial meniscus is attached to the medial collateral ligament and is more commonly injured.

49 The leg is divided by fascia lata into anterior, lateral and posterior compartments. The anterior compartment contains the extensors of the toes and dorsiflexors of the ankle joint (tibialis posterior, extensor hallucis longus, extensor digitorum longus and peroneus tertius). They are supplied by the deep branch of the common fibular nerve and the anterior tibial artery. The lateral compartment contains muscles that evert the subtalar joint complex and plantar flex the ankle (peroneus longus and brevis). Tibialis anterior inverts the foot, and peroneus longus has an important role in supporting the transverse arch of the foot. Damage to the common fibular nerve as it winds round the head of the fibula causes 'foot drop'.

50 There are two layers of muscles in the posterior (flexor) compartment of the leg; they have very important functions in gait and posture as well as being essential for normal venous return from the lower limbs. The superficial muscles (gastrocnemius, plantaris and soleus) are plantar flexors of the ankle and have a common powerful tendon, (tendo calcaneus or Achilles tendon), that attaches to the calcaneus. They are supplied by the tibial nerve and artery. Contractions of gastrocnemius and soleus assist the return of venous blood from the lower limbs (calf muscle pump). The tendons of the deep layer of muscles (popliteus, tibialis posterior, flexor digitorum longus, flexor hallucis longus) pass posterior to the medial malleolus with the tibial artery and nerve. Tibialis posterior plantar flexes and inverts the foot. Flexor hallucis longus inserts into the terminal phalanx of the big toe and is vital in the final push-off for running.

51 The foot supports the entire body weight and provides an elastic but stable platform for movement. A series of bony arches spread the body weight and act as shock absorbers. The arches are maintained partly by the pull of tendons, partly by bones locking into position when they are weight bearing and partly by powerful ligaments. The ankle joint (tibia, fibula and talus) is a stable hinge that allows *only* plantar flexion and dorsiflexion. The capsule and the collateral ligaments are strong but frequently sprained, particularly on the lateral side. Fractures around the ankle are common, but the joint rarely dislocates. There are a number of other joints in the foot that allow rotational movements between tarsals, metatarsals and phalanges. The joints are complex and involve multiple articular surfaces of the talus, calcaneus and navicular. Eversion is brought about by muscles in the lateral compartment of the leg, supplied by superficial fibular nerve (peroneus longus and brevis). Muscles attached to the medial side of the foot (tibialis anterior, tibialis posterior, extensor hallucis longus) supplied by the tibial nerve bring about inversion.

52 You do not need a very detailed knowledge of the anatomy of the foot; it is less often damaged than the hand. Recall the similarities of the sole of the foot to the palm of the hand. Superficially, the sole is protected by thick skin and dense fatty superficial fascia. The plantar aponeurosis provides the elastic component of the longitudinal arch. It is very dense and can hamper attempts to control bleeding from the plantar arch. The deep plantar arch and deep branch of the lateral plantar nerve lie deep to the flexor tendons with their four lumbrical mucles and flexor accessorius. The deepest plane includes the tendons of peroneus longus, tibialis posterior and interossei. The medial plantar nerve is similar in distribution to the median nerve and the lateral plantar is similar to the ulnar nerve in the hand.

53 Clinical testing of the nerve roots L_1–S_4 involves the examination of the myotomes, dermatomes and tendon reflexes of the lower limb for clinical signs of damage. The distribution of dermatomes differs from that in the upper limb because, during development, the lower limb rotates medially bringing the big toe into the midline, causing the dermatomes to spiral around the limb. Peripheral nerves arising from the lumbosacral plexus are tested by their cutaneous distribution.

Head and neck

54 The skull is complex but can be considered as two compartments: the cranium and facial skeleton. The cranium consists of flat bones joined by fibrous suture joints. The frontal bone forms the anterior part of the cranium. Paired parietal and temporal bones form the lateral and superior surfaces and a single occipital bone lies posteriorly enclosing the foramen magnum. Nodding movements occur between the occipital condyles and the atlas vertebra (C1). The bones of the face are irregular and easily damaged, particularly around the orbit; the maxillae and ethmoid bones are hollow, enclosing the paranasal air sinuses. The only synovial joint in the skull is the temporomandibular joint between the head of the mandible and the temporal bone. At birth, the bones of the cranium are not fully formed and are connected by fibrous membranes (anterior and posterior fontanelles). Because the mastoid process and tympanic plate of the temporal bone develop after birth, the facial nerve and eardrum are superficial and vulnerable to damage in the newborn.

55 The anterior cranial fossa houses the frontal lobes of the brain. The temporal lobes occupy the middle cranial fossa. The greater wing of the sphenoid makes up the floor of the middle fossa in which there are important foramina for vessels and cranial nerves. In the midline, the body of the sphenoid forms the pituitary fossa. The petrous temporal bone separates the middle and posterior cranial fossae. The occipital bone forms the floor of the posterior cranial fossa, encloses the foramen magnum and supports the cerebellum, pons and medulla. The brain and spinal cord are covered by the meninges. Pia mater is the deepest layer and is closely applied to all the complex folds on the surface of the brain. The larger arteries and veins of the brain lie between the pia and the arachnoid mater in the subarachnoid space, which is filled with cerebrospinal fluid. Dura mater is the tough inner lining of the cranium that encloses the dural venous sinuses and forms folds such as the tentorium cerebelli, which physically support the brain.

56 Sympathetic neurones that supply structures in the head or neck arise in the lateral grey columns of the spinal cord between T_1 and T_2. Preganglionic fibres that supply structures in the head synapse in the superior cervical sympathetic ganglion and are carried on the internal carotid artery and its branches to the orbit and skin. Sympathetic stimulation causes vasoconstriction, sweating and dilatation of the pupil. Levator palpebrae superiores is partially supplied by sympathetic nerves. The 12 cranial nerves are numbered in the order they arise from the brainstem. They leave the cranium via named foramina in the base of the skull. Some are entirely sensory (olfactory, optic and vestibulocochlear), some are entirely motor (trochlear, abducens, accessory and hypoglossal). Four carry parasympathetic fibres (oculomotor, facial, glossopharyngeal and vagus). The others are mixed.

57 The right common carotid artery arises from the brachiocephalic trunk. The left common carotid artery arises directly from the aortic arch. Both pass upwards on either side of the trachea enclosed in the carotid sheath with the internal jugular vein and vagus nerve. The common carotid arteries give no branches in the neck and divide at C3 into the external and internal carotid arteries. The external carotid supplies structures in the neck and face and terminates as the maxillary and superficial temporal arteries. The internal carotid gives no branches in the neck and enters the skull through the carotid canal, carrying sympathetic fibres on its wall. The artery has a tortuous course before terminating as the anterior and middle cerebral arteries. Posteriorly, the brain is supplied by the vertebral arteries that arise from the first part of the subclavian artery. They travel in the foramina transversaria of cervical vertebrae to reach the foramen magnum and join to form the basilar artery. This supplies the posterior parts of the brain and communicates via the Circle of Willis with the internal carotid artery.

58 Blood from the brain drains to a number of dural venous sinuses, which eventually empty into the internal jugular vein at the jugular foramen. The internal jugular vein joins with the subclavian vein, which drains the upper limb, to form the brachiocephalic vein at the root of the neck. The brachiocephalic veins unite to form the superior vena cava. The maxillary and superficial temporal veins join within the parotid gland to form the retromandibular vein. The posterior auricular and retromandibular veins drain into the external jugular, which empties into the subclavian vein. The subclavian vein is the most anterior structure, lying on the 1st rib just behind the middle of the clavicle; it is commonly used for the insertion of central venous lines.

59 The scalp receives a rich blood supply from branches of the internal and external carotid arteries. The skin of the scalp, underlying connective tissue and aponeurosis of occipitofrontalis are firmly linked and move freely on the deeper loose areolar tissue overlying the pericranium. The facial artery crosses the lower border of the mandible at the anterior edge of masseter. Facial skin is supplied entirely by the ophthalmic, maxillary and mandibular divisions of CN V. The muscles of facial expression are supplied by branches of CN VII, which lies within the

parotid gland. The parotid gland is a large salivary gland wedged between the angle of the mandible and the mastoid process. Its duct crosses masseter, pierces buccinator and opens into the vestibule of the mouth. The retromandibular vein, auriculotemporal nerve and the terminal part of the external carotid artery all pass through the parotid. The gland is supplied by parasympathetic neurones that travel with a branch of CN IX, synapse in the otic ganglion and are distributed by the auriculotemporal nerve.

60 There are four muscles of mastication: masseter, temporalis, lateral and medial pterygoids. They are all supplied by the motor root of CN V. Movements associated with chewing take place at the temporomandibular joint. A large, fibrocartilagenous disc divides the cavity into two separate compartments. During relatively small movements (talking), the disc is stationary and the head of the mandible moves within the concavity of the disc. When the mouth is opened widely, the head of the mandible *and* the disc move forwards together and the movement occurs between the disc and the temporal bone. The infratemporal fossa lies deep to the ramus of the mandible in front of and beneath the temporal bone. The fossa contains the lateral and medial pterygoid muscles surrounded by the pterygoid venous plexus. The external carotid artery terminates as the superficial temporal and maxillary arteries within the fossa; the most important is the middle meningeal branch of the maxillary artery, which is at risk in fractures of the pterion. The mandibular division of CN V and its motor root enter the fossa from the foramen ovale above.

61 The eyelids consist of loose skin, the tarsal plates and the circularly arranged muscle fibres of obicularis oculi, which blink the eye. Levator palpebrae superioris, which lifts the upper eyelid, is partly formed of smooth muscle supplied by sympathetic nerves. The cornea is protected by the conjunctiva. Blinking spreads tears across the conjunctiva from lateral to medial; excess drains into the nasolacrimal sac and duct, which open into the inferior meatus of the nasal cavity. The orbit contains the eyeball, optic nerve, ophthalmic artery and its branches, and the extraocular muscles and their cranial nerve supply. The extraocular muscles move the eyeballs to coordinate their gaze. The four recti are attached to a tendinous ring posteriorly, forming a cone by attaching to the sclera just behind the cornea. The two oblique muscles reach the eyeball from the bony wall of the orbit. Five of the extraocular muscles are supplied by CN III. This nerve also carries preganglionic parasympathetic fibres to supply the constrictor pupillae and ciliary body. Dilator pupillae is supplied by sympathetic fibres.

62 The mouth extends from the lips to the palatoglossal fold immediately anterior to the tonsils. The roof consists of the hard and soft palates and the floor is formed by the tongue and the mylohyoid muscle. The tongue is muscular and it may slip back into the pharynx to block the airway in unconscious patients. The tongue is supplied by the lingual artery and is drained by the lingual vein, a branch of the external carotid. The dorsum is divided into an anterior two-thirds, which receives common sensory innervation from the lingual nerve (CN V_c) with taste fibres from the chorda tympani, and a posterior one-third, which is innervated by the pharyngeal plexus (CNs IX and X). The submandibular gland lies under the mandible with the lingual artery curving around it. Its duct passes forward close to the lingual nerve and opens into the floor of the mouth. The sublingual glands lie along the submandibular duct. Both glands receive a parasympathetic secretomotor supply via the chorda tympani fibres (CN VII) carried by the lingual nerve.

63 The pharynx lies posterior to the nose, mouth and larynx, forming the upper portions of the digestive and respiratory tracts. Its wall consists of superior, middle and inferior constrictor muscles, which pass inferiorly and laterally from the posterior raphe to attach to their various bony insertions. The major features of the nasopharynx are the opening of the auditory tube, the tubal tonsil and the naospharyngeal tonsil. Behind the mouth and anterior to atlas and axis, the oropharynx contains the palatine tonsils. The laryngopharynx is the common passage for the digestive and respiratory tracts. It lies between the epiglottis and the beginning of the oesophagus at C6. The innervation of the pharynx is by the pharyngeal plexus (CNs IX, X and XI) with some sympathetic fibres. Swallowing is a complex process that involves raising the larynx towards the hyoid and the base of the tongue; this results in the epiglottis flipping downwards to cover the laryngeal inlet. The process is controlled by CNs VII, IX, X, XI and XII.

64 The nasal cavities form the upper part of the airway and extend from the nostrils to the choanae posteriorly. The lateral walls consist of the maxilla, ethmoid, three conchae and the palatine bones. The median nasal septum rarely lies exactly in the midline. The floor consists of the hard palate and the roof is formed by the cribriform plate, through which pass the branches of CN I. The frontal, maxilla, ethmoid and sphenoid bones are hollow and lined by respiratory epithelium, forming the paranasal air sinuses. The larynx is a complex three-dimensional structure. It consists of a series of articulating hyaline cartilages connected by fibroelastic membranes. The vocal folds stretch across the lumen in the median plane between the arytenoid and cricoid cartilages at the level of C4 (just below the laryngeal prominence) and, with the arytenoid cartilages, form the glottis. Immediately above the true vocal folds are false vocal folds, which lie at the inferior margin of the vestibule. The larynx performs three

major functions: phonation, control of the glottic aperture and control of the inlet during swallowing. Branches of CN X nerve provide both sensory and motor innervation.

65 The neck consists of five columns. The bony muscular column comprises the cervical spine, surrounded by muscles and enclosed by prevertebral fascia. The visceral column comprises the pharynx/oesophagus, larynx/trachea and the thyroid gland enclosed by pretracheal fascia. There are two neurovascular bundles, each surrounded by the carotid sheath containing the common and internal carotid arteries, internal jugular vein, the vagus nerve and the cervical chain of lymph nodes. Finally the entire neck is enclosed by deep investing fascia, wrapped around like a collar. The posterior triangle of the neck is formed by sternocleidomastoid, trapezius and the middle part of the clavicle. The triangle contains the trunks of the brachial plexus, the apex of the lung, the spinal part of the accessory nerve, the cervical plexus C_1–C_4, the subclavian artery and some groups of lymph nodes.

66 The boundaries of the anterior triangles are the anterior border of sternocleidomastoid and the midline and lower border of the mandible. Superficially within the triangles are the infrahyoid strap muscles. Deep to them is the trachea: the continuation of the larynx below the cricoid cartilage at C6. Posterior to the trachea, the oesophagus is the continuation of the pharynx with the carotid sheaths on either side. The thyroid is an endocrine gland that secretes thyroid hormones (thyroxine and triiodothyronine) and calcitonin. It consists of two lobes lying on either side of the trachea linked anteriorly by the isthmus, which lies in front of tracheal rings 2–4. The gland is attached to the trachea by pretracheal fascia and it moves with the larynx and trachea during swallowing. It receives a rich blood supply from the external carotid and thyrocervical trunk of the subclavian artery. Venous drainage is to the internal jugular and the brachiocephalic veins. The recurrent laryngeal nerves (CN X) lie in the groove between the oesophagus and trachea, closely related to the inferior thyroid artery. The external laryngeal nerve is accompanied by the superior thyroid artery.

67 The wall of the eyeball has three layers: the outer tough layer of sclera and cornea, the middle layer of vascular choroid posteriorly and the ciliary body (iris and the ciliary processes) anteriorly, and the inner coat. The inner coat has two layers: one that is reflective and one that forms the deepest part of the eyeball containing the light-sensitive rods and cones. The ciliary body divides the eye into two chambers: the anterior chamber lying between cornea and iris and the posterior chamber between iris and lens and containing aqueous humour. The lens lies behind the iris and is attached to the ciliary processes by the suspensory ligament. Behind the lens the eye is filled with vitreous humour. The optic nerve is covered by the meninges as it travels in the optic canal to the middle cranial fossa and the optic chiasm. The central vein of the retina is vulnerable to raised intracranial pressure as it passes through the subarachnoid space to drain into the ophthalmic veins.

The structure of the ear is very complex, with outer, middle and inner portions. The outer ear consists of the pinna (or auricle), the external acoustic meatus and the tympanic membrane, which completely separates the outer and middle ears. The ossicles (malleus, incus and stapes) span the middle ear cavity and transmit sound vibrations between the tympanic membrane and the inner ear. The cavity is connected directly to the nasopharynx and is prone to infection; consequently, the internal carotid artery and the facial nerve, which are intimately related to it, are at risk. The inner ear is a closed hydraulic system entirely encased within the petrous temporal bone. It is concerned with the senses of hearing and balance (CN VII).

68 For each cranial nerve, there are tests that will determine if its function is impaired. These tests examine both motor and sensory functions.

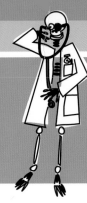

Fleshed out

There is a lot of anatomy and it is difficult to know where to start and sometimes where to stop! In the chapters that follow you will find a succinct review of core material and plenty of diagrams to help you to begin to visualize the most important structures. As you build up your knowledge, you will also find it useful to look at more realistic illustrations and a photographic atlas of anatomy. It is worth remembering that anatomical accounts may sometimes seem to divide structures rather arbitrarily into different regions; for example, structures from the upper limb, neck and thorax will be mentioned in the root of the neck where all three regions converge. When you are studying these linking regions, use the index to find cross-references to other parts.

1. Anatomical terms

Questions
■ What is meant by 'the anatomical position'?
■ What are the three basic planes of the body?

In common with other professions, medical practice requires the use of a very extensive technical language. Many terms are derived from Latin or Greek and you should begin to notice that the beginnings and ends of words recur frequently; if you understand their meanings, it will certainly help you to learn them (see the Glossary). As a starting point, you should be able to understand and use the following anatomical words appropriately.

Basic positional terms

Basic positional terms relate to the **anatomical position** (Fig. 3.1.1), body standing upright, arms hanging down with the palms forward (and penis erect!). Remember that these terms apply even when a patient is lying down.

superior (**cephalic**)	**inferior** (**caudal**)
nearer head	nearer feet
anterior (**ventral**)	**posterior** (**dorsal**)
nearer front	nearer back

proximal nearer to the root of the structure	**distal** further from the root of the structure
superficial nearer to the skin	**deep** further from the skin
ulnar medial side of forearm	**radial** lateral side of forearm
palmar anterior surface of hand	**dorsum** posterior surface of hand
tibial medial side of leg	**fibular** lateral side of leg
plantar inferior surface of foot	**dorsum** superior surface of foot

Phrases such as 'the brachial plexus is closely **related** to the axillary artery' means that the plexus lies in close physical proximity to the artery. It follows, for example, that we can talk about the **anterior relations** of the artery, meaning structures that lie anteriorly. Relations are important when you are trying to understand what the effects of trauma could be or how disease processes spread.

Basic planes

Basic planes (Fig. 3.1.2) are important when describing computed tomographic scans (CAT). Look at the sections of the head to understand these terms.

Median means in the middle: a plane that divides the body into two equal halves right and left; **medial** is nearer to the

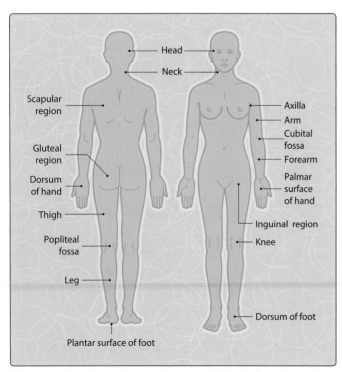

Fig. 3.1.1 Anterior and posterior views of the body to show the anatomical position and anatomical regions.

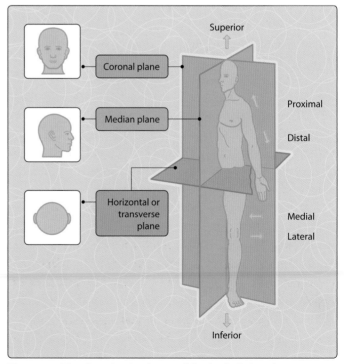

Fig. 3.1.2 The three basic planes of the body (related to magnetic resonance imaging of the head).

median plane, **lateral** is further from the median plane. Terms such as superolateral or inferolateral are used as intermediates (like northwest or northeast).

Sagittal planes are parallel to the median plane.

Coronal planes are at right angles to the median plane.

Movements

Movements provide important descriptive terms for physical examination.

flexion folds a joint

extension straightens a joint

dorsiflexion pulls the foot up at the ankle

plantiflexion pushes the foot down at the ankle

abduction away from the median plane

adduction towards the median plane (*adds* your arm to your side)

ulnar deviation adduction at the wrist

radial deviation abduction at wrist

rotation where part of the body rotates on its own longitudinal axis (shaking of head)

pronation rotation of the palm of hand posteriorly

supination carries the palm anteriorly and helps you to carry your *soup* bowl

inversion turns the foot inwards

eversion turns the foot outwards

Adduction and abduction of the fingers and toes are movements towards and away from the median plane of the hand and foot (in the plane of the nails). The movements of the thumb, however, are described differently because the metacarpal of the thumb is rotated through 90 degrees to the plane of the fingers. Abduction of the thumb carries it anteriorly away from the palm and adduction carries it posteriorly towards the palm.

Surface anatomy

Clinical procedures and physical examinations of patients require an accurate understanding of the structures under the skin and the ability, with the aid of landmarks, to visualize the outline of those structures on the skin. These important landmarks are referred to as **surface markings**. They are often bony landmarks (e.g. in the gluteal region, the sciatic nerve lies midway between the ischial tuberosity and the greater trochanter of the femur).

A good way to learn this aspect of anatomy is to use your own body ('they can't take that away from you!'). Bony landmarks can either be seen or be palpated through the skin. Take every opportunity to observe normal anatomy at rest or in action. Analyse what you see in pictures of sporting activities. Observe the changes that occur within the lifespan of individuals. Your

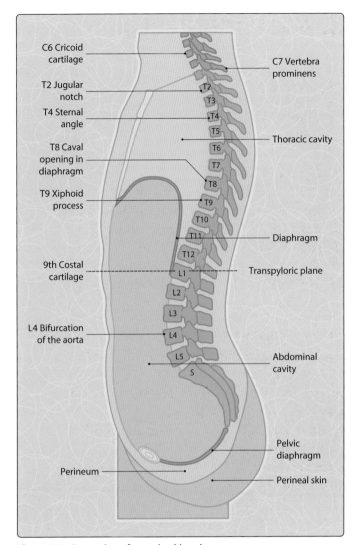

Fig. 3.1.3 Examples of vertebral levels.

growing knowledge will ensure that you will be able to recognize the unusual or abnormal. It is always interesting to consider what structures would be damaged in a stab wound of a particular region, or which structures your needle would pass through if you were required to perform a biopsy.

Vertebral levels and cross-sectional anatomy

In clinical practice, the horizontal level of a structure is sometimes described in relation to the vertebra at the same level. This is known as the **vertebral level** of a structure, e.g. the sternal angle lies at T4 and marks the bifurcation of the trachea (Fig. 3.1.3 and Table 1.1). Horizontal levels are particularly important when you are looking at CT or MRI scans. These scans are often cross (transverse) sections of the body. Cross-sectional images can be challenging to interpret because you have to apply your knowledge in a different dimension.

2. The vertebral column

Questions
- What are the boundaries of the intervertebral foramen?
- What is meant by a slipped disc?
- What movement occurs at the atlanto-axial joint?

The vertebral column protects the spinal cord, provides support for the skull and confers flexibility through the articulation of 33 individual vertebrae. It is divided into five regions (Table 3.2.1), with the vertebrae of each region modified from a basic plan (Fig. 3.2.1) for the functional needs of that region. The **body** of the vertebra is the weight-bearing component. The bodies increase in size from the head down and contain red bone marrow throughout life, which is supplied by a network of vessels

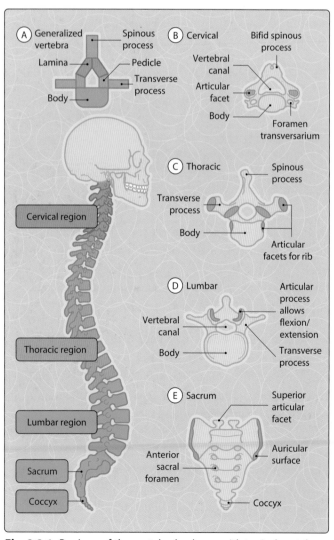

Fig. 3.2.1 Regions of the vertebral column with typical vertebrae.

including vertebral, intercostal and lumbar arteries. Venous drainage is to the azygos system (p. 69).

The **neural arch** encloses the vertebral canal. It consists of two pedicles and two laminae. The pedicles are notched above and below to form the boundaries of the intervertebral foramina, through which all the spinal nerves emerge (Fig. 3.3.2, p. 30). The **spinous process** projects posteriorly and inferiorly and two **transverse processes** project laterally. There are two **superior** and two **inferior articular facets** for the facet (zygapophyseal) joints between adjacent vertebrae (Fig. 3.2.3).

Vertebral joints
The vertebrae are held together by intervertebral joints, facet joints and longitudinal ligaments. The intervertebral joints between the bodies of the vertebrae (Fig. 3.2.2) are specialized cartilaginous joints consisting of an outer, tough mesh of interlacing fibres, the **annulus fibrosus**, which holds in place the resilient **nucleus pulposus**, which acts as a shock absorber. The shape of the two synovial facet joints governs the movement between the individual vertebrae. Arthritic changes are associated with these joints.

The longitudinal ligaments form a tube linking all the elements of the vertebrae: anterior and posterior **longitudinal ligaments** connect the bodies, **interspinous** and **supraspinous ligaments** link the spinous processes and the **ligamentum flavum** connects the laminae.

The muscles of the abdominal wall, psoas and quadratus lumborum cause flexion and lateral flexion of the column while normal upright posture (requires extension of the vertebral column) is brought about by postvertebral muscles (erector spinae group), which arise from the vertebrae and insert into the ribs.

Characteristics of specific vertebrae
The **atlas** and **axis** are cervical vertebrae specialized to form the connection to the head. The atlas (C1) articulates with the occipital condyles of the skull on either side of the foramen magnum. The **atlanto-occipital joint** allows nodding and lateral flexion of the head. The atlas has no body. The transverse processes are large and can be palpated in the neck immediately behind the angle of the jaw.

The body of the atlas fuses with the axis (C2) during development to form the dens (odontoid process). The dens articulates with the anterior arch of the atlas forming the **atlanto-axial** joint around which the head pivots when you shake your head. There are 'mission critical' ligaments that support this joint (rupture would result in the spinal cord being crushed!). Radiographs of these joints are usually taken through the open mouth.

There are two important surface landmarks. **C7** is the **vertebra prominens**, normally the first palpable spinous process. **L3/L4 junction** is determined by a line joining the highest points of the iliac crests and is the usual site for lumbar puncture (p. 31).

PROLAPSE OF AN INTERVERTEBRAL DISC

The nucleus pulposus lies closer to the posterior part of the disc and age-related degeneration or traumatic damage to the annulus fibrosus may allow the nucleus to prolapse: a 'slipped disc' (Fig. 3.2.3). The nucleus may compress either the spinal cord or the roots of spinal nerves, giving neurological symptoms (e.g. compression of sacral nerves may give rise to **sciatica**).

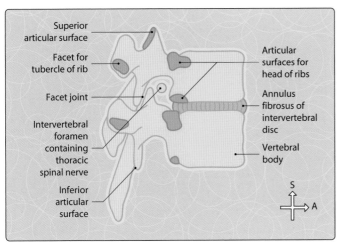

Fig. 3.2.2 Lateral view of an intervertebral foramen showing the relationships of the spinal nerve.

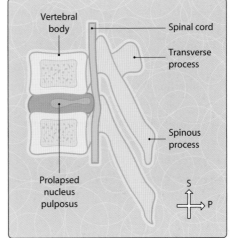

Fig. 3.2.3 Section of thoracic vertebrae showing prolapse of an intervertebral disc.

Table 3.2.1 CHARACTERISTICS OF VERTEBRAE OF REGIONS OF THE BACK

Region	Unique features	Functional aspects	Curves
Cervical (7)	Small bodies, large triangular vertebral canal, foramina transversaria for the vertebral arteries (p. 138), bifid spinous processes; atlas and axis articulate with head	Most mobile region; supports skull and vertebral arteries *Movements*: flexion, extension, lateral flexion, rotation	Secondary develops at 3 months, when a baby can lift its head; lordosis
Thoracic (12)	Heart-shaped body, long spinous processes, long transverse processes, facets for articulation with ribs (p. 54)	Articulations with ribs allowing respiratory movements *Movements*: rotation	Primary present at birth; kyphosis
Lumbar (5)	Very large body, transverse processes short and strong	Weight bearing, facets prevent rotation *Movements*: flexion, extension, latera flexion	Secondary develops when a child begins to walk; lordosis
Sacral (5)	Vertebrae are fused in adults; articulates at the sacroiliac joints; supported by the sacroiliac ligaments	Sacroiliac joint attaches pelvic girdle to the vertebral column *Movements*: very limited	Primary present at birth; kyphosis
Coccygeal (3–5)	Fused variable	*Movements*: none	

Lordosis, concave posteriorly; kyphosis, concave anteriorly.

3. Spinal cord and spinal nerves

Questions
- Why is it important to understand dermatome patterns?
- At what level does the spinal cord terminate in an adult?

The **central nervous system** (CNS) consists of the brain and spinal cord. The **peripheral nervous system** consists of the cranial and spinal nerves and the autonomic nervous system. The autonomic nervous system consists of a parasympathetic and a sympathetic division; these control involuntary activities (see Fig. 1.1).

Although the original pattern is lost during formation of the brain and cranial nerves, the arrangement of the cord and spinal nerves still reveals that they are derived from embryonic segments (somites). Each segment of the spinal cord gives rise to a pair of spinal nerves. As they emerge from the intervertebral foramina (p. 29), they are numbered according to the adjacent vertebra. There are 8 cervical, 12 thoracic, 5 lumbar, 5 sacral and 1 coccygeal spinal nerves (Fig. 1.4).

Spinal cord

At an early stage of fetal development, the spinal cord extends the whole length of the vertebral canal. However, since the vertebral column grows more quickly than the spinal cord, by the time a baby is born the cord only reaches as far as L3. This differential growth continues during childhood and by adulthood, the cord ends at the level of L1/L2. This gradual retreat upwards of the terminal part of the cord means that, although cervical spinal nerves arise close to their own intervertebral foramen and have a short course within the canal, lumbar and sacral nerves have to travel down the vertebral canal for some distance before they reach their correct exit point (e.g. spinal nerve L$_1$ will pass downwards from its origin and emerge from the intervertebral canal between L1 and L2). Below L1/L2, the canal does not contains the spinal cord but a collection of descending nerve roots known as the **cauda equina** (horse's tail) (Fig. 3.3.1).

The meninges that cover the brain (p. 134) also enclose the spinal cord (Fig. 3.3.2) and the subarachnoid space is filled with cerebrospinal fluid (CSF). The pia mater continues beyond the end of the cord as the **filum terminale**, which attaches to the coccyx. The arachnoid and dura mater end at S2.

Spinal nerves

Spinal nerves are described as mixed nerves. The **dorsal root** carries **sensory fibres** from the peripheral sense organs *to the* spinal cord. The **ventral root** carries both **motor fibres** being carried *from* the spinal cord to effector organs and **sympathetic**

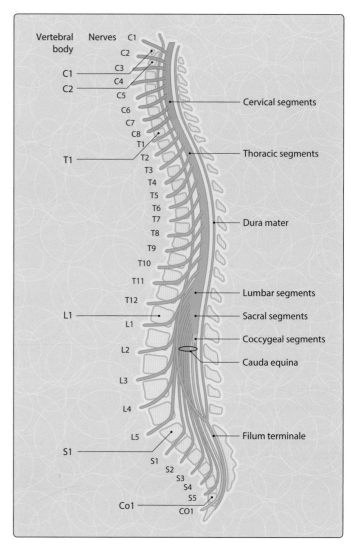

Fig. 3.3.1 Lateral view of the adult spinal cord within the vertebral canal showing the course of spinal nerves within the vertebral canal.

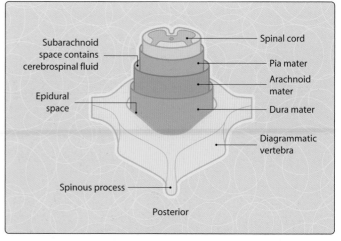

Fig. 3.3.2 Step dissection of the spinal cord and its meninges.

preganglionic fibres travelling to adjacent sympathetic ganglia. The sympathetic ganglion is connected to the spinal nerve via the white and grey rami communicantes. Sympathetic ganglia are the sites of synapses between the cell bodies of pre- and postganglionic cells (Fig. 3.3.3). The spinal nerves divide to form the:

- **dorsal ramus** supplying the erector spinae muscles and the skin that overlies it
- **ventral ramus** supplying the muscles and skin of the remaining body wall.

The blood supply of the spinal cord is complex and obviously it is critically important that it is not interrupted. Superiorly, the cord is supplied by longitudinal anterior and posterior spinal arteries, branches of the vertebral arteries as they enter the foramen magnum. The rest of the cord is supplied by segmental arteries such as the cervical, intercostal and lumbar arteries, which enter the cord through the intervertebral foramina. The venous drainage is also segmental and without valves; consequently, the veins communicate freely with one another. They drain first into the **internal vertebral venous plexus**, which lies in the epidural space, and then into the external venous plexus, which also drains the bodies of the vertebrae. Blood is finally carried into the azygos system of veins that lie on the posterior thoracic wall.

Plexus formation and root values

The limbs are supplied by groups of spinal nerves that combine to form a plexus. The brachial plexus comprises spinal nerves supplying the upper limbs (p. 40). The lumbar and sacral plexuses supply the lower limbs (p. 110). Subsequent branching patterns ensure that named nerves carry fibres from more than one spinal segment and that each spinal segment contributes to more than one named nerve. The spinal segments that contribute to a named nerve are known as its **root value**. It is useful to know the root values of important nerves in order to perform neurological examinations. The biceps reflex jerk tests the musculocutaneous nerve that has a root value of C_5, C_6, C_7. Failure to elicit the reflex suggests a problem either with the musculocutaneous nerve itself or, more seriously, with the spinal segments that contribute it.

Dermatomes

A dermatome is a strip of skin supplied by a single spinal segment (Fig. 1.3). Sensitivity of the skin is easy to test and may give important clues to the level of nerve damage but patterns are variable and the areas of the dermatomes overlap considerably.

Myotomes

A group of skeletal muscles that are supplied by a single spinal segment is known as a myotome, e.g. the small muscles of the hand are supplied by T_1. Knowledge of dermatome distribution and myotomes is important when investigating damage to the spinal cord or spinal nerves.

LUMBAR PUNCTURE

The spinal cord terminates at L2; below this level the vertebral canal is filled by lumbar and sacral spinal nerves as they seek to exit via their own intervertebral foramina. Between L1 and S2, these nerves are enclosed by dura and arachnoid mater (the lumbar cistern). A needle can safely be inserted below the level of the cord at L3/L4, to sample CSF. This procedure is known as lumbar puncture and may be performed to investigate infection of meninges (meningitis). During surgical procedures in the pelvis and perineum, anaesthetics can be injected into the extradural or subarachnoid space at L3/L4 to achieve epidural or spinal anaesthesia of those spinal roots that form the cauda equina.

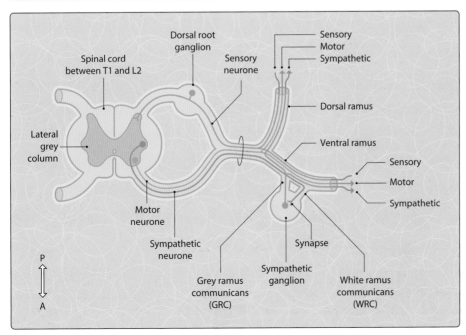

Fig. 3.3.3 Cross-section of the thoracic spinal cord showing the connection to a sympathetic ganglion and the composition of a spinal nerve.

4. Bones of the upper limb

Questions
- Why is the clavicle more likely to fracture than to dislocate?
- Which bones are most likely to be damaged in a fall on the outstretched hand?

The pectoral girdle, which attaches the upper limbs to the trunk, consists of the scapulae and clavicles. It does not form a complete bony ring like the pelvis because there is no joint with the vertebral column (Fig. 3.4.1). Posteriorly, the limbs are suspended by muscles that are attached to the vertebrae.

Clavicle (collar bone)

The clavicle acts as a strut that increases the range of abduction at the **glenohumeral (GH) joint** by supporting the limb in a lateral position (Fig. 3.4.2). It articulates medially with the sternum at the **sternoclavicular joint**, which is the *only* bony attachment of the upper limb to the trunk and is very effectively

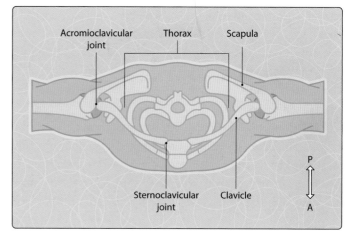

Fig. 3.4.1 Cross-section of the thorax showing the attachment of the pectoral girdle.

stabilized by strong ligaments and an intra-articular disc. Laterally, the clavicle articulates with the acromion of the scapula at the **acromioclavicular (AC) joint**. The clavicle transmits

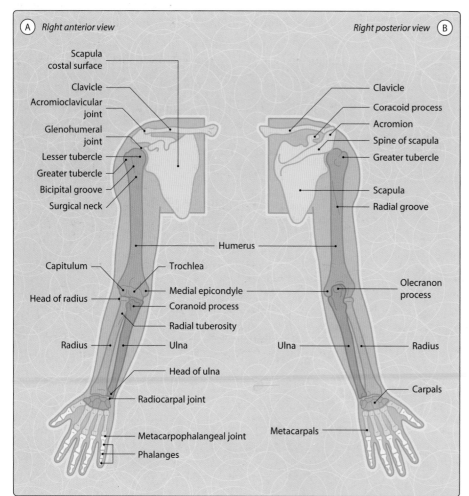

Fig. 3.4.2 Bones of the right upper limb. (A) Anterior view; (B) posterior view.

forces from the arm to the sternum; because it is supported at both ends by strong ligaments, it is more likely to fracture than to dislocate.

Scapula (shoulder blade)

The scapula is a flat triangular bone that provides attachment for a number of powerful muscles. The clavicle articulates with the acromion at the AC joint and is the most lateral bony point of the shoulder region. The AC joint is stabilized by strong ligaments that fix the coracoid process to the inferior surface of the clavicle (see Fig. 3.9.1, p. 42). Laterally, the **glenoid fossa** provides a shallow socket for the head of the humerus to form the GH joint. The spine of the scapula normally lies at the level of the spinous process of T3 and the inferior angle lies at T8 (or the seventh rib posteriorly).

Humerus

The **head** is hemispherical, but at any time only one-third of its surface can articulate with the glenoid fossa at the GH joint (p. 42). The head is connected to the shaft by the **anatomical neck**, which is thickened by the greater and lesser tubercles to provide attachment for the rotator cuff muscles (p. 42). Between the tubercles is the bicipital (intertubercular) groove for the tendon of the long head of biceps. Inferior to the tubercles, the shaft narrows to form the **surgical neck**, a common site of fracture. The axillary nerve lies in direct contact with the bone of the surgical neck and is vulnerable to damage in a fracture or dislocation of the GH joint.

Posteriorly, there is a shallow spiral groove, the radial groove, where the radial nerve lies in contact with the bone. Distally, the **capitulum** articulates with the head of the radius and the **trochlea** with the ulna.

Radius and ulna

The complex articulations between the humerus, radius and ulna permit flexion and extension at the elbow and **pronation and supination** of the forearm (Fig. 3.4.3). In the supinated position, the palm of the hand faces anteriorly and the radius and ulna lie parallel. During pronation, the radius (carrying the hand) pivots around the ulna and the forearm bones cross. The olecranon process of the ulna is the bony point of the elbow (the funny bone). The ulnar nerve lies between the olecranon and the medial epicondyle of the humerus (Fig. 3.4.2); it is stimulation

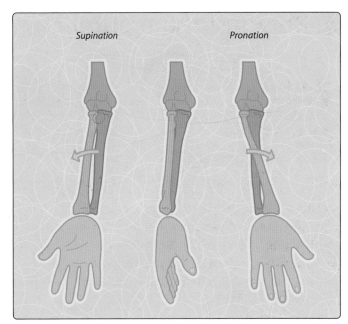

Supination   *Pronation*

Fig. 3.4.3 Relative position of the forearm bones in pronation and supination.

of this nerve that causes the unpleasant tingling sensation (paraesthesia) when you 'bang your elbow'. Distally, the radius articulates with the scaphoid and lunate to form the **radiocarpal joint**. The ulna does not articulate directly with the carpus; it is separated by a fibrocartilagenous disc that binds the radius and ulna together.

Carpus, metacarpals and phalanges

See p. 48.

 COMMON FRACTURES TO THE UPPER LIMB

When we trip, we automatically stretch out an arm to protect ourselves. The upper limb will often, therefore, take the full force of a fall. Depending on the nature of the fall, the force may result in fractures to:

- first metacarpal (Bennett's fracture, which may also involve the trapezium)
- scaphoid (tenderness in the 'anatomical snuff box')
- radius (Colles' fracture causes a 'dinner fork' deformity, which is a typical injury in osteoporotic patients)
- shaft of the humerus (at the surgical neck or spiral groove)
- middle third of clavicle (most commonly fractured bone).

5. Muscles of the outer chest wall and the axilla

Questions
- Which muscles bring about movements of the scapula on the thorax wall?
- Which muscles bring about abduction of the glenohumeral joint?
- What causes winging of the scapula?

The only **bony** attachment of the upper limb to the trunk is through the sternoclavicular joint; the powerful muscles of the chest wall attach the limb to the trunk. These can be divided into the muscles of the anterior chest wall (Fig. 3.5.1) and those of the back and shoulder (Fig. 3.5.2).

Muscles of the anterior chest wall

Pectoralis major arises from the sternum and clavicle and passes across the anterior chest wall, forms the anterior axillary fold and attaches to the bicipital groove of the humerus. It is a powerful adductor and flexor of the glenohumeral (GH) joint and is supplied by the lateral and medial pectoral nerves.

Pectoralis minor attaches the coracoid process of the scapula to the ribs (medial pectoral nerves).

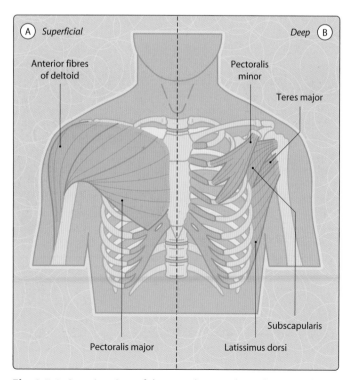

Fig. 3.5.1 Anterior view of the muscles attaching the upper limb to the thorax: (A) superficial muscles; (B) deep muscles.

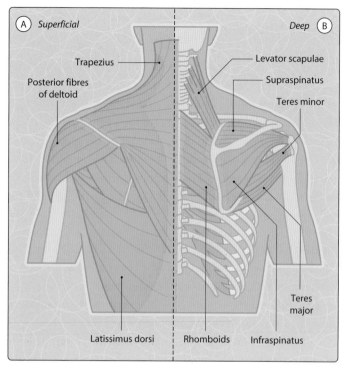

Fig. 3.5.2 Posterior view of the muscles attaching the upper limb to the thorax: (A) superficial muscles; (B) deep muscles.

Muscles of the back and shoulder

The powerful muscles of the back and shoulder region attach the pectoral girdle and upper limb to the axial skeleton (skull and vertebral column).

Superficial muscles of the back

Trapezius attaches the clavicle and spine of the scapula to the skull and the cervical and thoracic vertebrae. It elevates, retracts and helps to rotate the scapula laterally, and it stabilizes the pectoral girdle when carrying a heavy weight. It has an unusual nerve supply from cranial nerve XI (p. 136) because it has an attachment to the skull.

Latissimus dorsi arises from the lower thoracic and lumbar vertebrae and the iliac crests and inserts to the floor of the bicipital groove. It is a powerful adductor of the GH joint and can lift the whole body weight when climbing or performing a 'chin up' at the gym. It is supplied by the thoracodorsal nerve.

Deep muscles of the back

Rhomboid major and minor lie deep to trapezius and attach the medial border of the scapula to the thoracic vertebrae and retract the scapula. They are supplied by the dorsal scapular nerve.

Levator scapula attaches the medial border of the scapula to the cervical vertebrae and elevates the scapula; it is supplied by the dorsal scapular nerve.

Serratus anterior (sometimes called the boxer's muscle) is attached laterally to the upper eight ribs and to the medial border of the scapula. It pulls the scapula anteriorly, rotates it when the arm is raised above the head and also holds the scapula flat on the thorax wall when pushing forwards (protraction) or punching. It is innervated by the long thoracic nerve, which may be damaged during surgery. Loss of innervation allows the scapula to stick out when the patient pushes against something (winging of the scapula).

Short muscles of the shoulder

The short muscles of the shoulder attach the scapula to the humerus. They are important in stabilizing the GH joint.

Deltoid is attached proximally to the clavicle and spine of the scapula and inserts on to the lateral side of the humerus, giving the rounded shape to the shoulder. It is a powerful abductor of the humerus and stabilizes the GH joint when carrying a heavy load in the hand. Its anterior fibres flex, middle fibres abduct and posterior fibres extend the GH joint. It is supplied by the axillary nerve.

Teres major adducts and medially rotates the scapula; it is supplied by the lower subscapular nerve.

The four **rotator cuff muscles** are particularly important in stabilizing the GH joint (p. 43):

- **subscapularis**: arises from the anterior surface of the scapula and attaches to the lesser tubercle of the humerus
- **supraspinatus**: arises from the scapula above the spine and attaches to the top of the greater tubercle (assists abduction)
- **infraspinatus**: arises from the scapula below the spine and attaches to the greater tubercle
- **teres minor**: arises from the posterior aspect of the scapula and attaches to the greater tubercle.

Axilla

The pyramidal space between the thoracic wall and the upper part of the humerus is known as the axilla. Table 3.5.1 gives the boundaries of the axilla. Pectoralis major forms the anterior axillary fold and the muscles of the posterior wall form the posterior axillary fold. It contains the axillary lymph nodes and all the neurovascular structures passing between the neck and the limb; the nerves in particular are vulnerable to traction injuries of the neck (p. 53).

The axilla contains:

- structures lying between the outer border of the first rib and the inferior border of teres major, posterior to pectoralis major and pectoralis minor
- axillary artery and its branches
- axillary vein, lying medial to the artery
- cords and terminal branches of the brachial plexus arranged around the artery
- axillary lymph nodes.

Movement

The flexibility and range of movements of the arm are greatly increased by muscles that alter the position of the scapula on the thorax wall. These **scapulothoracic movements** (lateral and medial rotation, retraction and protraction, elevation and depression) are separate from the movements of the GH joint.

Table 3.5.1 BOUNDARIES OF THE AXILLA

Area	Boundaries
Apex	Clavicle, scapula, first rib
Anterior wall	Pectoralis major, pectoralis minor, clavipectoral fascia
Posterior wall	Subscapularis, teres major, latissimus dorsi
Medial wall	Serratus anterior, upper ribs
Lateral wall	Humerus
Base	Skin of the arm pit

RANGE OF MOVEMENT OF THE SHOULDER IN ARTHRITIS

The flexibility and range of movements of the shoulder are greatly increased by muscles that alter the position of the scapula on the thorax wall. These **scapulothoracic movements** (lateral and medial rotation, retraction and protraction, elevation and depression) are separate from the movements of the GH joint. Surprisingly, patients with very little abduction at the GH joint, as a result of severe arthritis, can still reach up to shelves by elevating their scapula.

6. Arterial supply

Questions
- Where are the arteries of the upper limb most vulnerable to damage?
- Where can the pulse be felt in the upper limb?
- Which arteries contribute to the blood supply of the hand?

The **subclavian artery** is the only arterial supply to the upper limb. The left subclavian artery arises as a direct branch of the arch of the aorta. The first branch from the arch is the brachiocephalic trunk, which divides posterior to the sternoclavicular joint to form the right subclavian and right common carotid arteries. The subclavian artery enters the axilla by crossing the first rib posterior to the subclavian vein and scalenus anterior muscle. In the neck, it gives a number of branches including the thyrocervical trunk,

which, in turn, branches to give the suprascapular and transverse cervical arteries. These pass posteriorly to supply the scapular region (Figs 3.6.1–3.6.3).

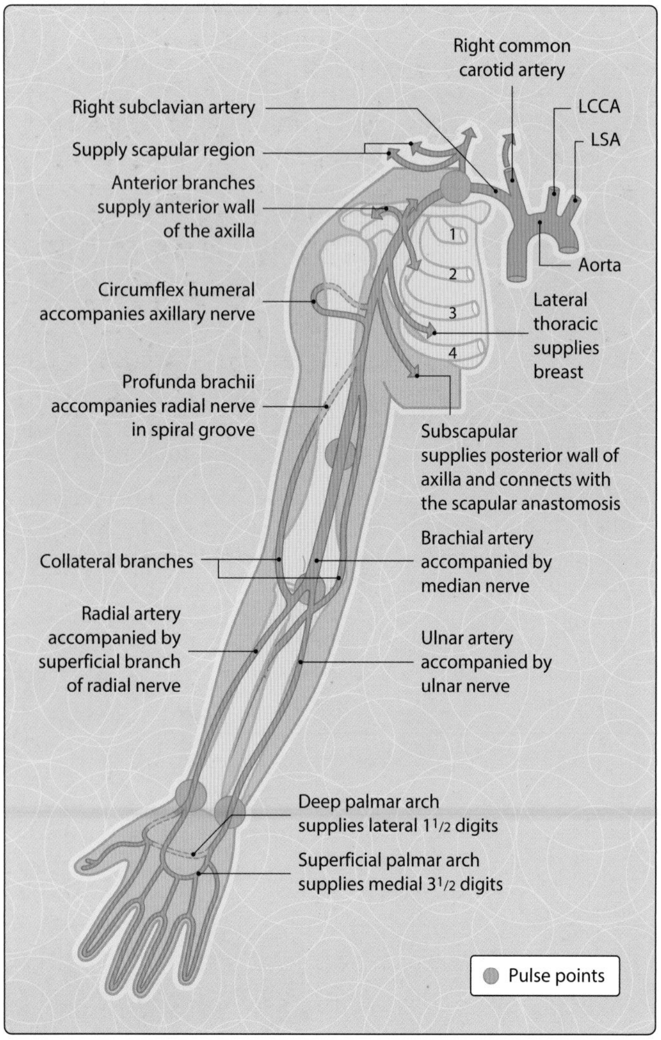

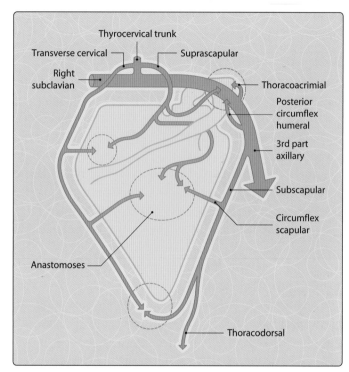

Fig. 3.6.2 Posterior view of right scapula to show the major areas of anastomosis between the subclavian and axillary arteries.

Fig. 3.6.1 Anterior view of the major arteries of the right upper limb.

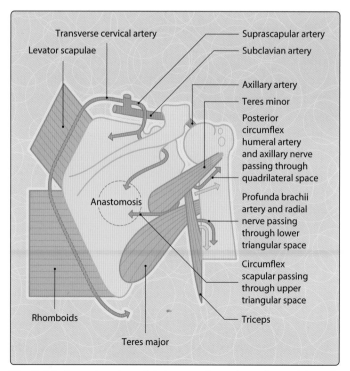

Fig. 3.6.3 Posterior view of right scapula to show the position of the major neurovascular structures.

Axillary artery

Beginning at the outer border of the first rib, the axillary artery passes posterior to pectoralis minor and is closely related to the cords of the brachial plexus (see Fig. 3.8.2, p. 40). Its branches supply the superior part of the thoracic wall, the muscular walls of the axilla and the lateral half of the breast. Its posterior branches connect with the branches of the subclavian artery supplying the scapular region, to form the **scapular anastomosis** (Figs 3.6.2 and 3.6.3). The axillary artery is closely related to the cords of the brachial plexus.

Brachial artery

The brachial artery begins at the inferior border of teres major as the continuation of the axillary artery. It lies in the anterior compartment of the arm accompanied by the median nerve and a pair of deep veins. It gives rise to the profunda brachii artery, supplying triceps, and collateral branches that anastomose around the elbow with branches of the ulnar artery. Anterior to the elbow joint, deep to the bicipital aponeurosis, the brachial artery terminates by dividing to form the **radial and ulnar arteries** (p. 44). The pulse of the brachial artery can be felt in the cubital fossa, *medial* to the biceps tendon and is located during the measurement of blood pressure.

Ulnar artery

The ulnar artery passes deep to the superficial flexor muscles of the forearm and gives the following branches:

- collateral branches, which contribute to the anastomosis around the elbow
- anterior interosseous, supplying the deep flexor muscles
- posterior interosseous, supplying the extensor compartment.

At the wrist, lateral to the pisiform bone, the artery passes superficial to the flexor retinaculum with the ulnar nerve. Just deep to the palmar aponeurosis and level with the distal border of the extended thumb, the ulnar artery forms the **superficial palmar arch**, which is usually completed by a small superficial palmar branch from the radial artery. The branches of the superficial arch supply the medial $3\frac{1}{2}$ fingers (p. 49).

Radial artery

The radial artery passes distally with the superficial branch of the radial nerve. The pulse can be felt over the distal radius. Here it gives a small branch to the superficial palmar arch and continues laterally around the base of the thumb, deep to the tendons of the anatomical snuff box. It passes into the palm through the muscles that lie between the first and second metacarpals, to form the **deep palmar arch** and gives branches to the lateral $1\frac{1}{2}$ digits (p. 49). The deep palmar arch is completed by the deep branch of the ulnar artery and lies at the level of the proximal border of the extended thumb. Metacarpal branches link the deep and superficial arches, ensuring a rich supply to the digits in any position of the hand.

 ROLE OF ANASTOMOSES IN PROTECTING THE BLOOD SUPPLY OF THE ARM FOLLOWING TRAUMATIC INJURIES

Arteries are most vulnerable where they are relatively fixed or very superficial. In the upper limb, for example, the subclavian artery is restricted by scalenus anterior muscle as it crosses the first rib. Trauma to the upper part of the thorax may damage the subclavian or the axillary arteries. However, the scapular anastomosis provides alternative routes for blood flow and so the limb is rarely completely ischaemic. Likewise, the rich anastomoses between the superficial and deep palmar arches in the hand protect the supply to the digits when a laceration at the wrist severs either the radial or the ulnar artery.

7. Venous and lymphatic drainage of the upper limb and the breast

Questions
- Why is it important to know the position of the superficial veins?
- Where are breast tumours most likely to spread?

Superficial veins

Because they are very commonly used for venepuncture, it is important to know the position of the superficial veins of the upper limb (Fig. 3.7.1).

The **cephalic vein** begins on the lateral side of the dorsal venous arch of the hand, crosses the tendons of the anatomical snuff box, remains superficial and eventually pierces deep fascia just inferior to the clavicle to join the axillary vein.

The **basilic vein** begins on the medial side of the dorsum of the hand and is usually connected to the cephalic vein anterior to the elbow by the **median cubital vein** (most common site for venepuncture). Just above the elbow, the basilic vein pierces deep fascia medially and joins with the deep veins to form the axillary vein.

The **axillary vein** lies within the curve of the axillary artery, receiving tributaries from the axillary and scapular regions. It lies anterior to scalenus anterior as it crosses the first rib and continues as the **subclavian vein** in the neck, before joining with the internal jugular vein to form the brachiocephalic vein (Fig. 3.7.1).

Deep veins

The deep veins are the **venae comitantes** that accompany major arteries.

Lymphatic drainage

All lymph from the upper limb and adjacent trunk above the umbilicus drains to the axillary nodes (Fig. 3.7.2). There

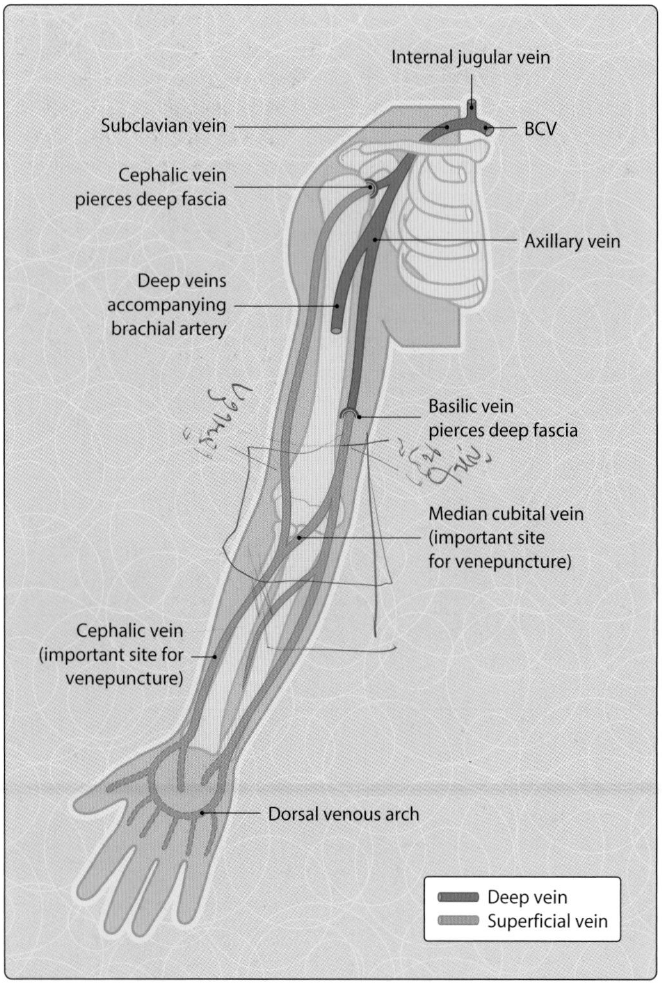

Fig. 3.7.1 Anterior view of the major veins of the right upper limb.

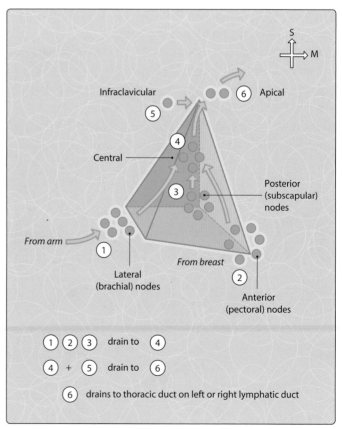

Fig. 3.7.2 Diagram to show the arrangement of lymph nodes in the right axilla.

Table 3.7.1 AXILLARY LYMPH NODES

Group	Location	Drains
1 Anterior/pectoral	Inferior border of pectoralis minor and the lateral thoracic vessels	Breast, thoracic and abdominal walls above the umbilicus
2 Lateral	Medial to axillary vein	Upper limb
3 Posterior/subscapular	Posterior axillary wall and the subscapular vessels	Scapular region and neck
4 Central	Embedded in axillary fat	Groups 1, 2, 3
5 Infraclavicular	Terminal part of the cephalic vein	Lateral part upper limb
6 Apical	Apex of the axilla	Groups 5 and 6

are six groups, totalling approximately 25–30 nodes in all (Table 3.7.1).

The axillary nodes drain via the apical group to the thoracic duct on the left and the right subclavian lymph trunk on the right. These lymph vessels then drain into the large veins at the root of the neck (usually at the point where the internal jugular and the subclavian veins meet).

■ THE BREAST

The anatomy of the breast and its lymphatic and venous drainage is important because in Western cultures 1 in 12 women will suffer from breast cancer (Fig. 3.7.3). The initial development of breast tissue in the superficial fascia of the chest wall is the same in both girls and boys. In girls, under the influence of oestrogen at puberty, glandular tissue differentiates and becomes embedded in fat. The breasts undergo further glandular development during pregnancy and secrete milk after the birth when stimulated by the hormone prolactin.

The medial part of the breast receives its arterial supply from the second, third and fourth perforating branches of the internal thoracic artery. The lateral half is supplied by thoracic branches of the axillary artery and there are deep branches from adjacent intercostal arteries. The venous drainage passes either anteriorly to the venae comitantes of the internal thoracic artery or to the posterior intercostal veins, which eventually drain to the azygos system (p. 69).

SPREAD OF BREAST CANCER

Approximately 75% of the lymph from the breast drains to the pectoral (anterior) group of axillary lymph nodes. Malignant cells may be carried in lymph vessels and undergo metastasis in the nodes of the axilla. Malignant cells can also be carried via intercostal veins to the azygos system and the vertebral venous plexus, causing secondary tumours in the thoracic vertebral bodies.

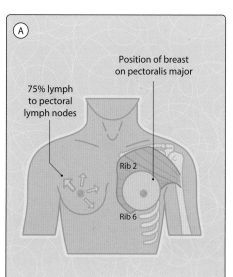

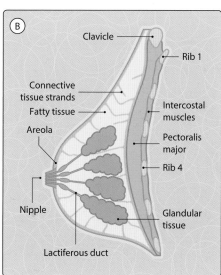

Fig. 3.7.3 The breast and its lymphatic drainage. (A) Anterior view; (B) sagittal section of the breast.

8. The brachial plexus

Questions
- Which of the trunks of the brachial plexus lies in contact with the first rib?
- Why can neck injuries or disease sometimes affect the function of the upper limb?
- Which of the terminal branches of the brachial plexus supplies the extensor compartments of the arm and forearm?

The brachial plexus originates from cervical spinal nerves (**ventral rami of spinal nerves C_5–T_1**) and supplies the skin and muscles of the upper limb (Fig. 3.8.1). The motor and sensory distribution of its nerves is reviewed on p. 52.

The brachial plexus is formed from the **ventral rami** of C_5–T_1, which combine to form three *trunks*, in the posterior *triangle* of the neck between the scalenus anterior and scalenus medius (p. 155). As the trunks cross the first rib posterior to the subclavian artery, the inferior trunk is in direct contact with the bone. Behind the clavicle, each trunk divides to form an **anterior** and a **posterior division**, which merge in the axilla to form **three cords**; these divide to form the important **terminal branches** (Fig. 3.8.2).

There are five terminal branches (Figs 3.8.3–3.8.6).

1. The **musculocutaneous nerve** (C_5–C_7) arises from the lateral cord and supplies the flexors of the elbow and skin on the lateral side of the forearm.

2. The **median nerve** (C_5–T_1) arises from branches of the medial and lateral cords. It accompanies the brachial artery and is the most medial neurovascular structure in the cubital fossa (p. 44). It supplies all the muscles of the flexor compartment with the exception of flexor carpi ulnaris and the medial half of flexor digitorum profundus. It passes deep to the flexor retinaculum to supply the thenar muscles, as well as skin of the lateral side of the palm and lateral $3\frac{1}{2}$ digits. It is vulnerable at the wrist and may be compressed in carpal tunnel syndrome.

3. The **ulnar nerve** (C_8, T_1) arises from the medial cord. It lies in the posterior compartment, passing posterior to the medial epicondyle of the humerus. It supplies the most medial forearm flexors and passes superficial to the flexor retinaculum with its artery. It innervates most of the intrinsic muscles of the hand as well as skin on the medial side of the palm and medial $1\frac{1}{2}$ digits. It is vulnerable to damage at the elbow and wrist.

4. The **axillary nerve** (C_5, C_6) arises from the posterior cord. It supplies the deltoid and the skin over deltoid. It is very closely related to the inferior aspect of the capsule of the GH joint and lies in direct contact with the surgical neck of the humerus. It may be damaged in dislocation of the GH joint and in fractures of the surgical neck.

5. The **radial nerve** (C_5–T_1) arises from the posterior cord. It lies in direct contact with the humerus in the spiral groove and supplies all extensor muscles and all posterior skin. It is vulnerable in mid-shaft fractures of the humerus.

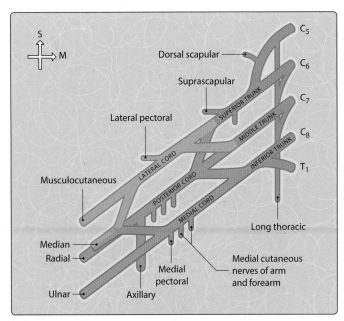

Fig. 3.8.1 Diagram of the right brachial plexus. Branches of the posterior cord supply the muscles of the posterior wall.

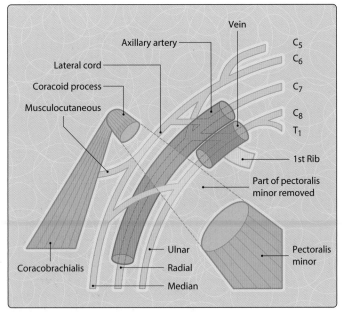

Fig. 3.8.2 Important relations of the right brachial plexus.

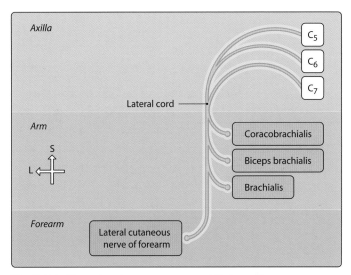

Fig. 3.8.3 Musculocutaneous nerve and its branches.

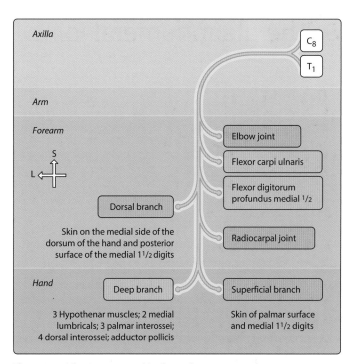

Fig. 3.8.5 Ulnar nerve and its branches.

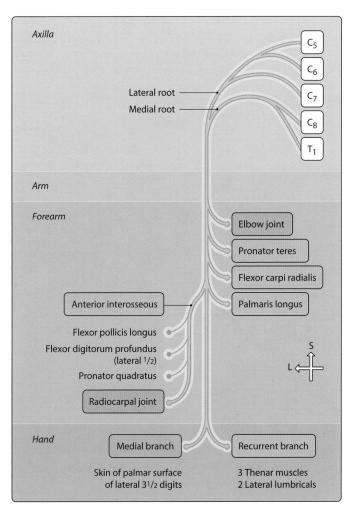

Fig. 3.8.4 Median nerve and its branches.

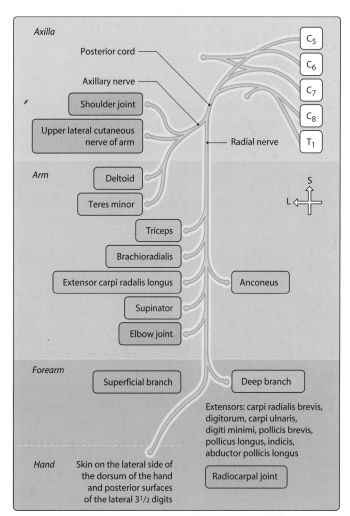

Fig. 3.8.6 Radial and axillary nerves and their branches.

9. The glenohumeral joint

Questions

- Why is the glenohumeral joint so unstable?
- Which three factors influence the stability of any synovial joint?
- Between which two structures does the subacromial joint lie?

The glenohumeral (GH) joint (Fig. 3.9.1) is relatively unstable; it is the most commonly dislocated large joint. It also has the greatest range of movement of any synovial joint.

Three factors influence the potential range of movement and stability of synovial joints:

- **bony contact**: the greater the contact between two articular surfaces, the more stable the joint will be (i.e. ball and socket joints like the hip are most stable)
- **ligamentous support**: ligaments develop in positions where they prevent unwanted movement at a joint (hinge joints like the elbow have strong lateral ligaments)
- **muscular support**: tendons that cross a joint will give support to the joint (e.g. the biceps tendon at the shoulder).

Movements

The GH joint allows movement around three axes; movements can be flexion (extension, abduction), adduction, rotation (medial and lateral) and circumduction. Abduction is a particularly free movement. It is widely suggested that the first 15° of abduction is brought about by the action of supraspinatus and movement continues to 90° under the influence of the powerful deltoid muscle; certainly both muscles are active in abduction. When the limb is stretched above the head, the scapula is rotated laterally by the action of serratus anterior and trapezius. It is important to distinguish between movement of the GH joint (i.e. between the head of the humerus and the glenoid fossa) and the movements of the scapula on the posterior wall of the thorax (scapulothoracic movements; p. 35).

The GH joint is poorly supported inferiorly and is particularly vulnerable in the abducted position, when it is prone to dislocate. In 80% of cases, the head comes to lie anteriorly, in the subcoracoid position. The characteristics of the articular surfaces, ligaments and muscles allow flexibility in movement and the tendency to dislocate.

Articular surfaces

The GH joint is more like an egg and spoon than a ball and socket. The head of the humerus is approximately hemi-

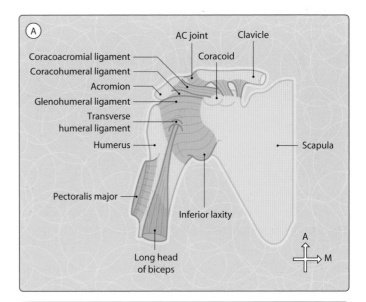

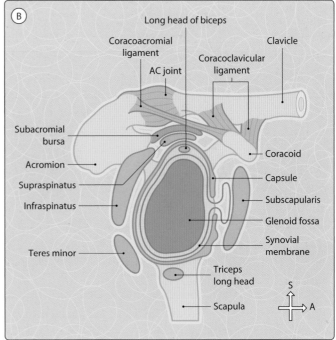

Fig. 3.9.1 The right glenohumeral joint. (A) Anterior view of the capsule; (B) lateral view of the capsule of the glenoid fossa (humerus removed).

spherical. The articular surface of the glenoid is very shallow and only accommodates about one-third of the humeral head at any time even though it is deepened by a fibrocartilagenous collar, the glenoid **labrum**.

We know that the labrum provides effective support because the joint is more prone to dislocation if the labrum is damaged.

Table 3.9.1 THE FOUR ROTATOR CUFF MUSCLES OF THE GLENOHUMERAL JOINT

SITS	Support glenohumeral joint	Additional action	Innervation
Supraspinatus	Superiorly	Initiates abduction	Suprascapular (C_5, C_6)
Infraspinatus	Posteriorly	Laterally rotates the humerus	Suprascapular (C_5, C_6)
Teres minor	Posteriorly	Laterally rotates the humerus	Axillary (C_5, C_6)
Subscapularis	Anteriorly	Medially rotates the humerus	Subscapular (C_5, C_6)

Capsule and ligaments

The ligaments provide support only anteriorly and superiorly (Fig. 3.9.1). The capsule is lax and is attached proximally to the margin of the glenoid labrum and distally to the anatomical neck of the humerus. It must be loose enough inferiorly to allow abduction of the humerus above the head; consequently, when the arm is adducted the capsule hangs in a fold. Anteriorly, the capsule is thickened to form a series of GH ligaments which prevent anterior dislocation. They act like the strings of a hammock: if one is torn, the support mechanism fails. Superiorly, the joint is supported by three structures. The **coracohumeral ligament** is a broad band that strengthens the capsule superiorly. The **tendon of the long head of biceps** lies in the bicipital groove of the humerus and is held in place by the **transverse humeral ligaments** between the greater and lesser tubercles. The tendon passes through an opening in the articular capsule to attach to the superior part of the glenoid fossa and acts like a guy rope over the joint. Within the capsule, the tendon is surrounded by a sheath of synovial membrane. Finally, the **coracoacromial ligament** forms an extremely strong arch between the acromion and the coracoid process. The ligament prevents superior dislocation of the humerus and adjacent bones are more likely to fracture than this ligament is to rupture.

Muscles

The four rotator cuff muscles, supraspinatus, infraspinatus, teres minor and subscapularis (SITS; Table 3.9.1) are very important in stabilizing the GH joint. **Subscapularis** arises from the anterior surface of the scapula and inserts into the lesser tubercle of the humerus (supplied by branches of the posterior cord of the brachial plexus). **Supraspinatus** arises from the scapula above the spine and attaches to the superior part of the greater tubercle (supplied by the suprascapular nerve). **Infraspinatus** arises from the scapula below the spine and attaches to the greater tubercle (supplied by the suprascapular nerve). **Teres minor** arises from the posterior aspect of the scapula and attaches to the greater tubercle (supplied by the axillary nerve).

These muscles form a musculotendinous cuff around the joint, protecting it and providing stability. The tone of the muscles is important. When contracted, they effectively hold the head of the humerus into the glenoid cavity. When relaxed the joint has greater freedom of movement. The inferior aspect of the joint is not supported by these muscles.

Tears in the rotator cuff tendons are common sports injuries where there is repetitive abduction of the joint (throwing, racquet sports). It can lead to degenerative tendonitis and irritation of the subacromial bursa (see below).

Bursae

There are a number of bursae associated with the GH joint. A bursa is a closed sac of synovial membrane containing a small amount of lubricating fluid. They are found either just under the skin or around tendons that are subject to friction. They allow skin to slide over an underlying bone (e.g. over the elbow and knee) or tendons to glide over bone in a restricted space without friction (e.g. flexor tendons at the wrist and in the fingers). The clinically most important bursa associated with the GH joint is the **subacromial bursa**. It occupies the very narrow space between the supraspinatus tendon and the coracoacromial arch (Fig. 3.9.1). If repetitive movements cause irritation of the bursa, it may become inflamed (bursitis) and damage the adjacent supraspinatus tendon, resulting in painful arc syndrome.

 CONSEQUENCES OF DISLOCATION OF THE GLENOHUMERAL JOINT

The GH joint is poorly supported inferiorly and is particularly prone to dislocate in the abducted position. Because the axillary nerve and its accompanying vessels are closely related to the inferior aspect of the capsule of the GH joint, they may be damaged, causing paralysis of deltoid and leading to loss of abduction and loss of sensation over the lateral aspect of the arm.

10. The arm, cubital fossa and elbow

Questions
- Which three nerves lie in direct contact with the humerus?
- Which nerve supplies the flexor compartment of the arm?
- What clinical procedures are performed in the region of the cubital fossa?

Anatomically, the arm is the upper limb from shoulder to elbow, not the whole limb (Fig. 3.10.1). The arm is divided by deep fascia into the anterior flexor and posterior extensor compartments (Fig. 3.10.1).

The flexor compartment

There are three muscles (BBC):
- biceps brachii is a powerful flexor of the elbow and supinator
- brachialis is a powerful flexor
- coracobrachialis flexes the GH joint.

The flexor compartment is supplied by the musculocutaneous nerve. Blood is supplied by the brachial artery and its branches.

The extensor compartment

The triceps muscle is the extensor of the elbow.

The extensor compartment is supplied by the radial nerve. Blood supply is via the profunda brachii artery.

Nerves

The **musculocutaneous nerve**, lying between biceps and brachialis, supplies the flexor compartment of the arm. The **radial** nerve, lying in the spiral groove, supplies the extensor compartment of the arm. The **median** nerve accompanies the brachial artery but gives no branches in the arm. The **ulnar** nerve lies medially but also gives no branches in the arm.

Three nerves lie in direct contact with the humerus and are vulnerable to damage (Fig. 3.10.2):
- axillary nerve: lies in contact with the surgical neck of the humerus (damage causes loss of abduction)
- radial nerve: lies in the spiral (radial) groove (damage causes wrist drop)
- ulnar nerve: lies between the medial epicondyle and the olecranon posterior to the elbow (damage causes claw hand).

Blood supply

The **brachial artery** is the continuation of the axillary artery in the arm (p. 37). Its pulsations may be felt against the shaft of the humerus in the groove on the medial side of the arm between the flexor and extensor muscles (Fig. 3.10.3). The brachial artery gives the following branches:
- **profunda brachii** artery, which passes posteriorly with the **radial nerve** (Fig. 3.6.1, p. 36) into the spiral groove on the posterior surface of the humerus

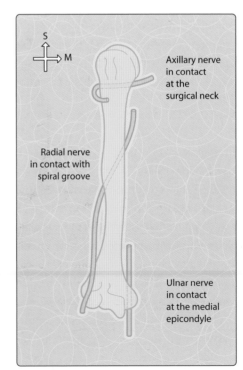

Fig. 3.10.2 The three nerves in direct contact with the humerus.

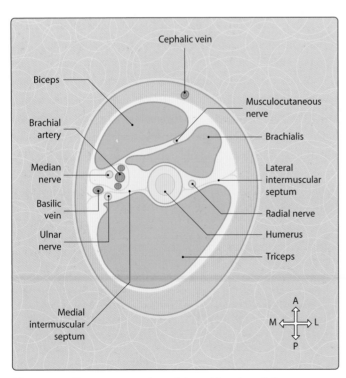

Fig. 3.10.1 Transverse section of the mid region of the arm.

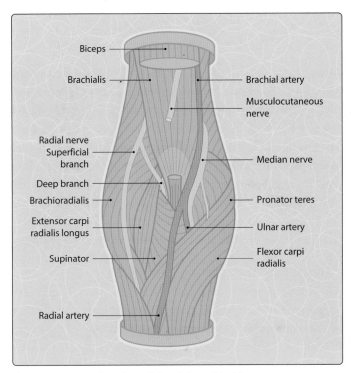

Fig. 3.10.3 Anterior view of the right cubital fossa.

Biceps
Brachialis
Brachial artery
Musculocutaneous nerve
Radial nerve Superficial branch
Median nerve
Deep branch
Brachioradialis
Pronator teres
Extensor carpi radialis longus
Ulnar artery
Supinator
Flexor carpi radialis
Radial artery

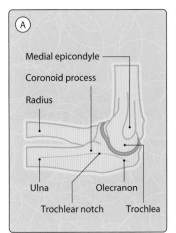
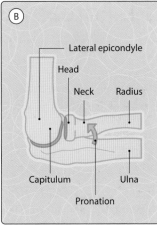

Fig. 3.10.4 The right elbow joint. (A) Medial view; (B) lateral view.

- **ulnar collateral branches**, which contribute to the anastomosis around the elbow joint.

The cubital fossa

The cubital fossa (Fig. 3.10.3) is a triangular depression in front of the elbow defined medially by pronator teres and laterally by brachioradialis. Contents of the fossa from medial to lateral are the median nerve, the brachial artery and the tendon of the biceps. The median cubital vein lies in the superficial fascia and is a common site for venepuncture. More deeply, the bicipital aponeurosis binds down and protects the median nerve and brachial artery as they pass anterior to the elbow joint. Blood pressure measurements are made over the brachial artery just medial to the biceps tendon.

■ THE ELBOW JOINT

The elbow joint (Fig. 3.10.4) is relatively stable in adults, but the joint and its adjacent structures are vulnerable to traumatic damage (think of those skate boarders!). The humerus, radius and ulna articulate within a single joint cavity. The capsule is lax in front and behind to allow a full range of flexion and extension. The collateral ligaments are strong and the joint is well supported by strong tendons. There are several possible movements.

- **Flexion and extension** of the elbow occur at the hinge joints between the capitulum and the head of the radius and between the trochlea and the trochlear notch of the ulna. Flexion is brought about by biceps and brachialis (musculocutaneous nerve), extension by triceps (radial nerve). The biceps tendon jerk tests spinal segment C_6 and the triceps jerk tests C_7.
- **Pronation and supination** occur at the **superior radioulnar joint** (pivot joint). Biceps is the most powerful supinator (musculocutaneous nerve) assisted by the supinator muscle and brachioradialis (radial nerve). During these rotatory movements, the ulnar remains almost stationary while the head of the radius rotates in the radial notch of the ulna, held in position by the annular ligament (supination helps you to hold your soup bowl!).

The inferior radioulnar joint lies at the distal end of the forearm bones (p. 32).

 PULLED ELBOW

The head of the radius rotates within the annular ligament during the movements of pronation and supination. The annular ligament attaches to the anterior edge of the radial notch of the ulnar, passes around the circumference of the head of the radius and attaches posteriorly to the notch. It is not attached to the radius but forms a collar that holds the head in position as it rotates. In adults this is a stable arrangement but in children the collar is loose and the head of the radius may be pulled out if a child is lifted or swung by one arm.

11. Forearm

Questions
- How does the ulnar nerve reach the forearm?
- What is the nerve supply of the flexor muscles of the forearm?
- Which of the carpal bones forms the floor of the anatomical snuff box?

Anatomically the forearm lies between the elbow and radiocarpal joints, with flexor and extensor compartments.

Flexor compartment

The flexor compartment contains the long flexors of the radiocarpal joint and digits, mostly supplied by the median nerve. There are two groups of muscles (Table 3.11.1):

- **superficial flexors** (Figs 3.11.1 and 3.11.2) arise from a common tendon attached to the medial epicondyle of the humerus; inflammation of the common flexor tendon gives rise to medial epicondylitis (golfer's elbow)
- **deep flexors** (Fig. 3.11.3) arise from the forearm bones and the interosseous membrane.

The vessels and nerves lie between the superficial and deep muscle layers. The ulnar nerve lies in the posterior compartment of the arm and passes posterior to the elbow joint between the olecranon and the medial epicondyle. It lies medial to the ulnar artery on the medial side of the forearm between flexor carpi ulnaris and flexor digitorum profundus. The radial nerve spirals round the humerus and crosses the elbow anteriorly on the lateral side of the cubital fossa; while its deep motor branch passes posteriorly to supply the extensors, the superficial branch accompanies the radial artery under cover of the brachioradialis muscle. The median nerve is the most medial structure of the cubital fossa and passes deep to the superficial muscles. At the level of the radiocarpal joint, it becomes superficial and lies between flexor digitorum superficialis and flexor carpi radialis.

Extensor compartment

The extensor compartment contains the extensors of the radiocarpal joint and digits, which are innervated by the termination of the radial nerve, the posterior interosseous nerve (Fig. 3.11.4):

- superficial group arises from a common extensor tendon originating on the lateral epicondyle of the humerus
- deep group arises from the forearm bones and interosseous membrane.

The muscles extend the wrist and digits and details of their attachments are given on p. 51. Inflammation of the common extensor tendon gives rise to lateral epicondylitis (tennis elbow).

The vessels and nerves that supply this compartment lie between the superficial and deep muscle layers. The muscles are innervated by the posterior interosseous nerve.

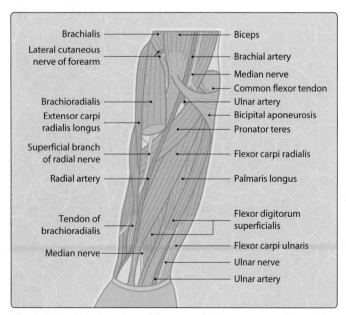

Fig. 3.11.1 Anterior view of the superficial structures of the right forearm. Middle portion of brachioradialis removed.

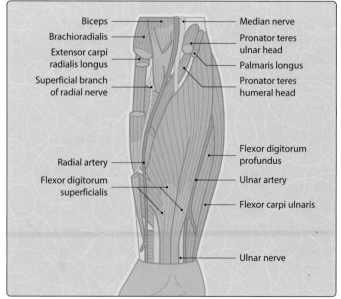

Fig. 3.11.2 Anterior view of the intermediate structures of the right forearm. Brachioradialis, extensor carpi radialis longus, pronator teres and palmaris longus removed.

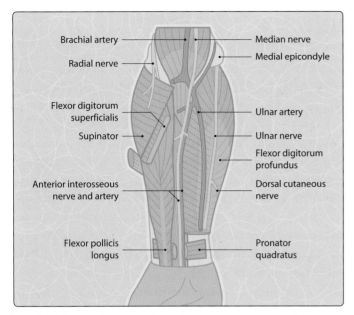

Fig. 3.11.3 Anterior view of the deep structures of the right forearm. Radial artery, superficial radial nerve, all superficial muscles and flexor digitorum superficialis removed.

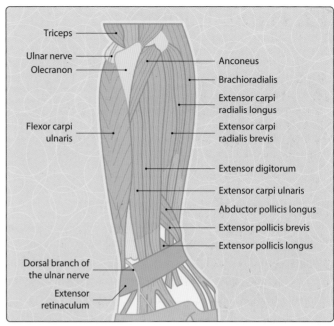

Fig. 3.11.4 Posterior view of the superficial structures of the right forearm.

The 'anatomical snuff box'

Extending and abducting the thumb demonstrates the 'anatomical snuff box': a hollow at the base of the thumb bounded laterally by the tendons of extensor pollicis brevis and abductor pollicis longus and posteriorly by the tendon of extensor pollicis longus (Fig. 3.11.4). On its floor, the scaphoid and the radial pulse can be palpated. Tenderness over this area suggests a fractured scaphoid. The superficial branches of the radial nerve and cephalic vein lie superficial to the tendons. It is a common site for venepuncture.

Table 3.11.1 THE SUPERFICIAL AND DEEP FLEXOR MUSCLES

Muscle	Action	Nerve
Superficial group		
Pronator teres (PT)	Pronation	Median
Flexor carpi radialis (FCR)	Flexion of radiocarpal joint and and abduction with extensor carpi radialis longus and extensor carpi radialis brevis	Median
Palmaris longus (PL)	Superficial, may be absent	Median
Flexor carpi ulnaris (FCU)	Flexion of radiocarpal joint and adduction with extensor carpi ulnaris	Ulnar
Flexor digitorum superficialis (FDS)	Four tendons attach to the middle phalanges of each finger gives flexion of MP and proximal IP joints (p. 50)	Median
Deep group		
Flexor digitorum profundus (FDP)	Four tendons: attach to the distal phalanges of each finger; flexion of MP and both IP joints (p. 50)	Lateral half by median[a] and medial half by ulnar
Flexor pollicis longus (FPL)	Flexion of MP and IP joints of the thumb	Median[a]
Pronator quadratus (PQ)	Pronation	Median[a]

[a]*Anterior interosseous branch.*
MP, metacarpophalangeal joint; IP, interphalangeal.

12. Hand 1: joints and movements

Questions
- Which bones make up the radiocarpal joint?
- What are the contents of the carpal tunnel?
- What are the functions of the thenar muscles and what is their innervation?

The radiocarpal joint and carpal tunnel

The distal radius articulates with the scaphoid and lunate to form the **radiocarpal joint** (Fig. 3.12.1). The head of the ulna is separated from the joint by a triangular fibrocartilagenous disc. The radiocarpal joint is stabilized by its capsule, strong collateral ligaments and the numerous tendons crossing it.

The carpus consists of eight small bones arranged in two rows bound by short ligaments. The carpal tunnel (Fig. 3.12.2) is formed by the **scaphoid, pisiform, trapezium** and **hamate** with the overlying deep fascia (flexor retinaculum). The proximal edge of the retinaculum lies deep to the distal skin crease at the wrist. The tunnel contains nine tendons and the **median nerve**; nerve compression leads to carpal tunnel syndrome (p. 53). (NB The ulnar nerve and artery are superficial to the flexor retinaculum.)

The flexor pollicis longus is surrounded by its own **synovial sheath** while the eight tendons of the flexor digitorum superficialis and the flexor digitorum profundus are enclosed by a common sheath. The extensor tendons are individually bound down to the posterior aspect of the radius and ulna by the extensor expansion (Fig. 3.12.3 and p. 51).

Movements of the digits

The hand is capable of powerful grips, which depend on the long forearm muscles, and fine precision movements, which involve the intrinsic (short) muscles of the hand. **Flexion** and **extension** of the fingers occurs at the metacarpophalangeal and interphalangeal joints. **Abduction** is movement away from the midline of the hand and **adduction** is towards the midline. Movements of the thumb differ because it is at 90° to the fingers (p. 27). **Opposition** is a complex movement involving rotation and flexion of the thumb, bringing it against the pad of any finger (Fig. 3.12.4).

Muscles

The **thenar eminence** is a group of three muscles at the base of the thumb. They arise from the adjacent carpal bones and insert on the metacarpal and proximal phalanx; they are innervated by the recurrent branch of the median nerve. **Abductor pollicis** and **flexor pollicis brevis** are superficial; **opponens pollicis** lies deep to the other two and is partly responsible for opposition of the thumb. **Adductor pollicis** also brings about fine movement of the thumb but is not part of the thenar group. It lies deeper in the palm attached to the third metacarpal. It is supplied by the

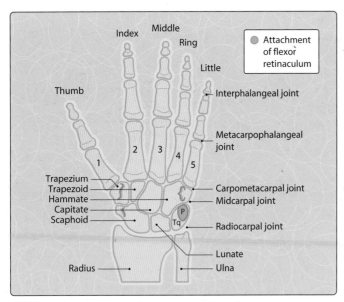

Fig. 3.12.1 Anterior view of the bones of the left hand. S, scaphoid; L, lunate; Tq, triquetrum; P, pisiform; Tm, trapezium; Td, trapezoid; C, capitate; H, hammate (remember as 'she looks terribly pretty, try to catch her').

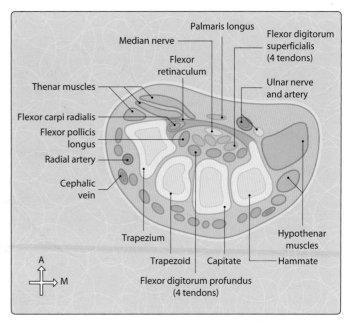

Fig. 3.12.2 Transverse section thorough the distal row of carpal bones showing the left carpal tunnel and its contents.

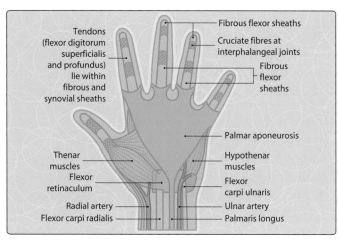

Fig. 3.12.3 Anterior view of the left hand to show components of the deep fascia and thenar eminence.

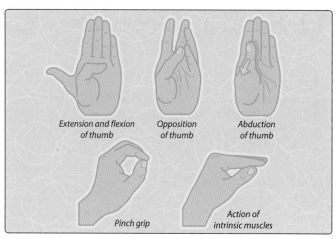

Fig. 3.12.4 Movements of the thumb.

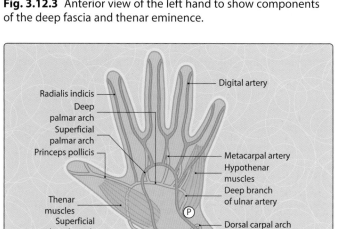

Fig. 3.12.5 Anterior view of the left hand to show the superficial and deep palmar arches.

deep branch of the ulnar nerve. The three **hypothenar muscles**, abductor, flexor and opponens digiti minimi, lie at the base of the little finger and are mirror images of the thenar muscles. They are supplied by the ulnar nerve.

The palm is complex (Table 3.12.1) and commonly damaged in falls and by lacerations.

Table 3.12.1 THE STRUCTURES IN THE PALM FROM SUPERFICIAL TO DEEP

Structure	Relationship in palm
Thick skin	Tightly bound down to deep fascia at the skin creases
Palmar aponeurosis	Protective sheet of deep fascia (Fig. 3.12.3) that attaches to metacarpals 3 and 5, dividing the palm into three fascial spaces that are important in the spread of infection
Superficial palmar arch	The continuation of the ulnar artery (Fig. 3.12.5) passes superficial to the flexor retinaculum, lateral to the pisiform; the arch lies at the level of the distal border of the extended thumb. Digital branches supply the medial $3\frac{1}{2}$ digits
Median and ulnar nerves	Motor and sensory branches
Flexor digitorum superficialis	Four tendons inserting into the middle phalanges
Four tendons of the flexor digitorum profundus	Inserting into the distal phalanges with four lumbrical muscles; the tendons of each digit are enclosed by fibrous flexor sheaths lined their synovial sheaths (Fig. 3.12.3 and Fig. 3.13.1, p. 50)
Four lumbrical muscles	From tendons of the flexor digitorum profundus; inserting into dorsal digital expansion
Deep palmar arch	The continuation of the radial artery (Fig. 3.12.4); lying deep to the tendons of flexor digitorum profundus at the level of the proximal border of the extended thumb; branches supply the lateral $1\frac{1}{2}$ digits and anastomose with the superficial arch
Ulnar nerve, deep branch	Supplies most of the intrinsic muscles of the hand
Adductor pollicis, three palmar and four dorsal interossei	Insert into the dorsal digital expansion

13. Hand 2: nerves and muscles

Questions
- What is the action of the intrinsic muscles of the hand?
- Which spinal segment gives the motor supply to the hand?

Long flexor tendons in the hand

From the distal forearm to their insertion on the phalanges, the tendons of the flexor digitorum superficialis (FDS) and flexor digitorum profundus (FDP) are surrounded by a common delicate **synovial sheath** that protects the tendons from damage (Fig. 3.13.1). Fibrous tunnels on the palmar surface of the phalanges hold the tendons close to the bones especially during flexion (Fig. 3.13.1). These fibrous flexor sheaths are thinner over the interphalangeal (IP) joints to allow flexion. In front of the proximal phalanges, the tendons of FDS split and insert into the sides of the middle phalanges, allowing the tendon of FDP to pass through and insert into the distal phalanx. The four **lumbrical muscles** arise from each of the tendons of FDP and insert into the dorsal digital expansions (see below).

Nerve supply and the intrinsic muscles of the hand

The small muscles that arise within the hand control its fine movements. They are innervated by T_1 fibres carried in the ulnar and median nerves. The considerable sensory supply is delivered by median, ulnar and radial nerves.

Median nerve

The median nerve (Fig. 3.13.2; see Fig. 3.12.2, p. 48) carries sensory impulses from the skin on the palmar surface of the lateral $3\frac{1}{2}$ digits and their nail beds. The motor supply goes to:

- three **thenar muscles** (see Fig. 3.12.3, p. 49): median nerve (recurrent branch) controls opposition of the thumb and other fine movements
- two **lateral lumbricals**: flex metacarpophalangeal (MP) and extend IP joints (Fig. 3.13.3).

If the median nerve is compressed in the carpal tunnel (carpal tunnel syndrome), fine control of thumb movements is impaired and there is tingling (paraesthesia) in the lateral $3\frac{1}{2}$ digits.

The ulnar nerve

The ulnar nerve deep branch (see Fig. 3.13.2 and Fig. 3.12.2, p. 48) carries sensory impulses from the skin on the palmar surface of the medial $1\frac{1}{2}$ digits and their nail beds. Motor supply is to the following intrinsic muscles:

- three **hypothenar muscles** (see Fig. 3.12.3, p. 49): opposition of the little finger and other fine movements
- two **medial lumbricals**: flex MP and extend IP joints

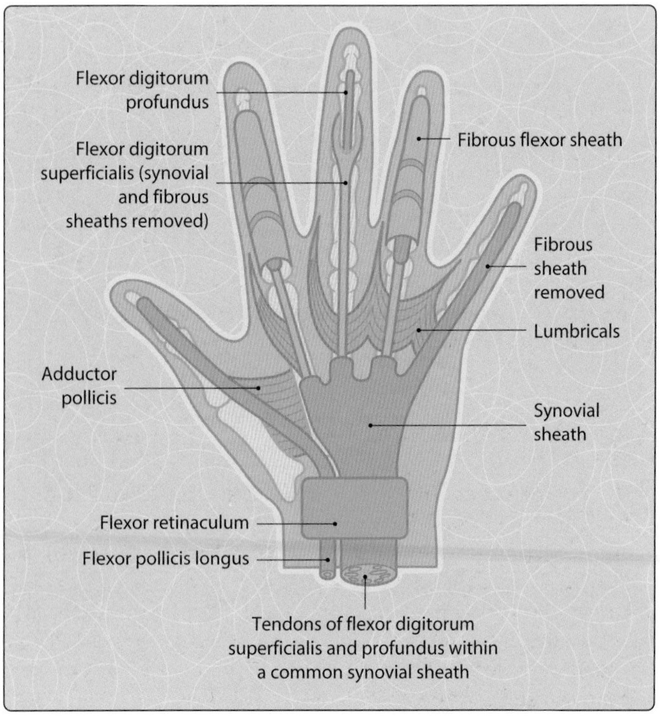

Fig. 3.13.1 Anterior view of the left hand showing the long flexor tendons with their fibrous flexor sheath and synovial sheaths.

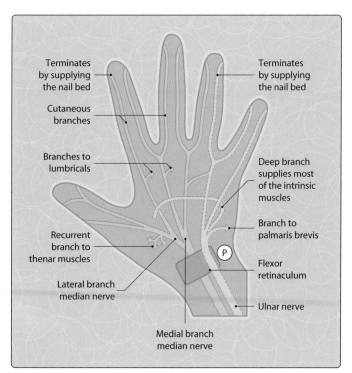

Fig. 3.13.2 Anterior view of the left hand showing the distribution of the median and ulnar nerves.

- three **palmar interossei**: <u>ad</u>duct the fingers (remember as PAD); flex MP and extend IP joints
- four **dorsal interossei**: <u>ab</u>duct the fingers (remember as DAB); flex MP and extend IP joints
- **adductor pollicis**: adduction of the thumb.

The radial nerve

The superficial branch of the radial nerve supplies skin on the lateral part of the dorsum of the hand and dorsal aspect of the lateral $3\frac{1}{2}$ digits. It gives no motor supply to muscles in the hand.

Back of the hand and the long extensor tendons

The thin skin of the back of the hand overlies the dorsal venous arch, which gives rise to the cephalic and basilic veins; they are important sites for venepuncture.

The extensor tendons are bound down to the wrist by the extensor expansion, where they are protected by short synovial sheaths. As the extensor tendons reach the posterior surface of the fingers, they flatten to form a triangular dorsal digital expansion (Figs 3.13.3–3.13.5). At its apex, the tendon splits and inserts onto the middle and distal phalanges (Fig. 3.13.4). The lumbrical muscles and interossei insert into the margins of the expansions. Extensor digitorum is unable to bring about extension of the IP joints without the synergistic action of the intrinsic muscles.

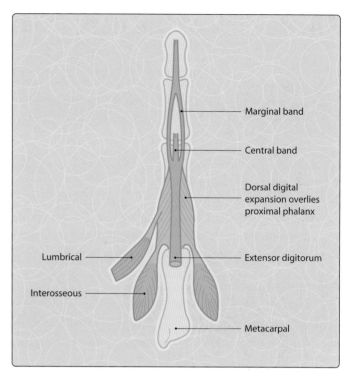

Fig. 3.13.4 Posterior view of the dorsal digital expansion and insertion of the extensor tendon.

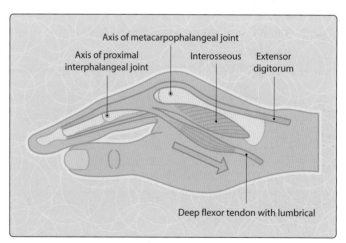

Fig. 3.13.5 Lateral view to show the relationship of the lumbricals and interossei to the metacarpophalangeal and interphalangeal joints.

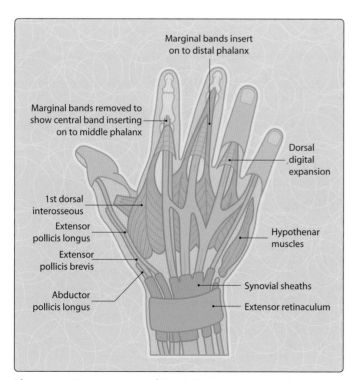

Fig. 3.13.3 Posterior view of the right hand showing the extensor tendons and dorsal digital expansion.

 ULNAR NERVE DAMAGE

The interossei and lumbrical muscles act together to flex the MP and extend the IP joints. If the ulnar nerve is damaged, for example by a laceration at the wrist, the intrinsic muscles are paralysed and the patient will develop a 'claw hand'. The long flexors cause flexion of the IP joints and the long extensors hyperextend the MP joints. This may seem to be a devastating injury; however, because the thenar muscles are intact, the hand can still perform a pinch grip.

14. Review of the nerve supply and clinical testing

Questions
- What nerve problems give rise to clinical signs in the upper limb?
- How do you test for nerve damage?

Problems related to the nerve roots of C_5–T_1 will give rise to clinical signs in the upper limb (Table 3.14.1). Clinical testing of these nerve roots involves the examination of the myotomes, dermatomes and tendon reflexes of the upper limb.

Motor distribution

The superior roots of the brachial plexus supply the most proximal part of the limb (C_5 and C_6 supply muscles that act on the shoulder) and the inferior roots supply the hand (T_1 supplies the intrinsic muscles of the hand).

Myotomes can be tested if spinal (central) damage is suspected by assessing movement:

C_5: abduction of the arm at the shoulder
C_6: flexion of the forearm at the elbow
C_7: extension of the forearm at the elbow
C_8: flexion of the fingers
T_1: adduction of the digits.

Sensory distribution

The distribution of the sensory nerves of the plexus is quite different from the motor distribution. Areas of skin on the limbs and trunk that are supplied by single spinal segments are known as **dermatomes**. The dermatomes of the upper limb are arranged in linear sequence around the central axis of the limb (p. 7). They are tested if spinal (central) damage is suspected.

Think of the dermatomes as a series of addresses to which fibres from a spinal segment are delivered. For example, think about the distribution of the cutaneous branch of the axillary nerve carrying C_5 and C_6 fibres. The C_5 fibres are preferentially delivered to the C_5 dermatome while the C_6 fibres are distributed more distally to the C_6 dermatome.

Test areas for dermatomes are:

C_5: over deltoid
C_6: tip of thumb
C_7: tip of index finger
C_8: tip of little finger
T_1: over the medial epicondyle.

Cutaneous distribution can also be described in another way. Each of the major nerves arising from the brachial plexus has cutaneous branches that supply a specific patch of skin (Table 3.14.2).

Brachial plexus lesions

The brachial plexus originates from cervical spinal nerves C_5–T_1. The trunks of the plexus lie in the posterior triangle of the neck and, therefore, may be damaged in penetrating injuries of the neck or if the head or upper limb is violently pulled away from the neck. For example, if the neck undergoes forced lateral

Table 3.14.1 SITES OF POSSIBLE NERVE DAMAGE

Site of damage	Nerve	Motor effect	Sensory loss
Shoulder dislocation	Axillary	Loss of abduction at the glenohumeral joint	Over deltoid
Fracture of surgical neck of humerus	Axillary	Loss of abduction at the glenohumeral joint	Over deltoid
Midshaft fracture of humerus or fracture of the neck of the radius	Radial (commonly only affects the posterior interosseous branch)	Inability to extend the wrist or digits (known as wrist drop)	Posterior skin of forearm and lateral side of the dorsum of the hand
Medial epicondyle humerus	Ulnar	Paralysis of the intrinsic muscles of the hand leads to a claw hand with hyperextended MP joints and flexed IP joints	Medial $1\frac{1}{2}$ fingers and ulnar border of the forearm
Carpal tunnel: compression of the contents (e.g. caused by swelling of synovial sheaths)	Median	Paralysis of thenar muscles leading to loss of fine control of thumb movements (particularly opposition)	Lateral $3\frac{1}{2}$ digits
Dislocation of lunate	Median	Paralysis of thenar muscles (see above)	Lateral $3\frac{1}{2}$ digits
Deep laceration at wrist	Median	Paralysis of thenar muscles (see above)	Lateral $3\frac{1}{2}$ digits

Table 3.14.2 CUTANEOUS DISTRIBUTION OF PERIPHERAL NERVES

Peripheral nerve	Cutaneous distribution
Axillary nerve	Skin over deltoid
Musculocutaneous	Terminates as the lateral cutaneous nerve of forearm
Median	Palmar surface of the lateral $3\frac{1}{2}$ digits
Ulnar	Palmar surface of the medial $3\frac{1}{2}$ digits
Radial	Posterior arm and forearm and the dorsal
Medial cutaneous nerve of arm (direct from medial cord)	Medial arm
Medial cutaneous nerve of forearm (direct from medial cord)	Medial forearm

flexion, the upper trunk (C_5, C_6) may be stretched or its roots may even be pulled out of the spinal cord. This type of injury will lead to paralysis of the muscles of the proximal part of the limb, which receive their supply from the upper trunk. The patient will be unable to abduct the shoulder, flex or extend either the shoulder or the elbow, and the limb will hang limply with the forearm pronated; there will be numbness down the lateral side of the limb over the C_5 and C_6 dermatomes. This injury sometimes results from motorcycle accidents and is known clinically as **Erb's paralysis**.

Similarly, damage to the lower trunk (C_8, T_1) occurs in forced abduction of the limb as sometimes occurs when an individual tries to break a long fall by hanging onto a support. Loss of T_1 results in paralysis of the intrinsic muscles of the hand and is known as **Klumpke's palsy**.

Damage to the motor supply of the diaphragm

It is important to remember that the motor supply to the diaphragm is mainly from C_4 the spinal segment, which lies immediately superior to those controlling the upper limb (C_5–T_1). Clinical testing of the upper limb will give important information in cases where there is concern that a neck injury may interfere with the control of breathing movements. Even in an unconscious casualty, tendon reflexes can reveal motor function of the spinal cord (e.g. biceps tendon tap tests for C_6 and triceps tests for C_7).

Damage to the radial nerve

The radial nerve may be damaged in fractures of the shaft of the humerus that involve the spiral groove. The motor branches to the three heads of triceps usually escape damage but the posterior interosseous nerve is affected and the patient will suffer from an inability to extend the wrist or digits. This will also affect the ability to form a tight grip (try to make a fist with a flexed wrist).

Carpal tunnel syndrome

The carpal tunnel contains the median nerve and the tendons of the long flexors of the digits. Synovial sheaths protect the tendons in this restricted space. Inflammation of the sheaths causes swelling, which may compress the median nerve, causing carpal tunnel syndrome. The symptoms include pins and needles (paraesthesia) over the thumb and lateral $2\frac{1}{2}$ fingers and weakness of the thenar muscles. Weakness of the thenar muscles is very troublesome as many activities depend on fine control of a pinch grip. In the long term, the thenar muscles will atrophy.

15. Thoracic cage

Questions
- What are the boundaries of the thoracic inlet?
- What are the attachments of the diaphragm?
- What is the thoracic level of the angle of Louis?

The embryo develops as a series of similar segments (somites). Each somite consists of a block of mesoderm that gives rise to voluntary muscle supplied by its own segmental nerve and artery. Postnatally, segmental structures are still recognizable in the organization of the body wall and particularly in the thoracic cage. Each thoracic segment consists of a vertebra, a pair of ribs and three layers of intercostal muscles supplied by segmental (intercostal) arteries and nerves (Figs 3.15.1 and 3.15.2).

The thoracic cage consists of:
- 12 pairs of ribs (Latin for rib, *costa*)
- 11 pairs of intercostal spaces (p. 56)
- the sternum
- 12 thoracic vertebrae with their intervertebral discs.

The thoracic cage protects the heart and lungs and overlaps some abdominal organs (e.g. liver and kidneys). The **inlet** of the thorax is a fixed bony ring formed by the vertebral body of T1, the first ribs (the 1st costal cartilage often ossifies during life) and

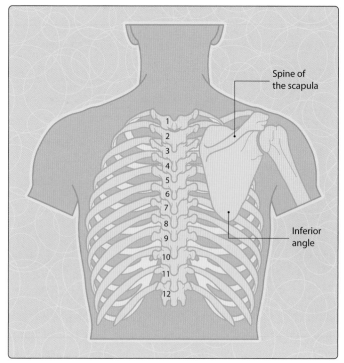

Fig. 3.15.2 Posterior view of the bony thoracic cage showing the position of the scapula.

the manubrium of the sternum. The diaphragm forms the thoracic **outlet** and is attached to vertebral body of T12, the 12th ribs, costal cartilages of ribs 7–12 (the costal margin) and the xiphisternal joint.

Ribs and costal cartilages
All the ribs have a head that articulates with thoracic vertebrae, a narrow neck, tubercle, shaft and costal cartilage (Fig. 3.15.3).

Typical ribs (3–10)
The **head** of a rib articulates posteriorly with the body of the same numbered vertebra, the body of the vertebra above and the intervening intervertebral disc. The **tubercle** of the rib articulates with the transverse process of the same numbered vertebrae and is marked by ligaments that support the joint (Figs 3.15.4 and 3.15.5). The angle is the weakest part of a rib. Rib fractures may result in a pneumothorax (p. 59).

The 12 ribs are divided into three groups in relation to their anterior articulation:
- ribs 1–7 (true ribs): articulate directly with the sternum via their costal cartilages
- ribs 8–10 (false ribs): their costal cartilages articulate with the adjacent costal cartilage above to form the costal margin
- ribs 11 and 12 (floating ribs): no articulation anteriorly.

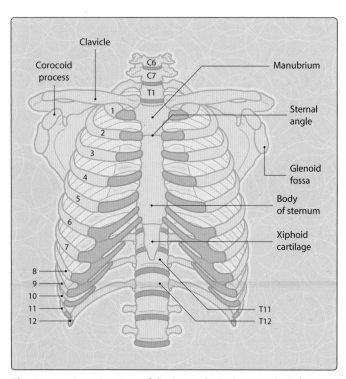

Fig. 3.15.1 Anterior view of the bony thoracic cage. Costal cartilages are shown in blue.

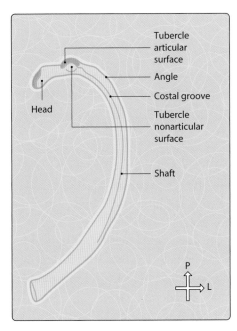

Fig. 3.15.3 View of a typical rib from above.

Ribs lie at an angle; the anterior part lies at a lower level to the posterior and so any horizontal section (e.g. CT and MRI scans) will cut through several ribs.

Atypical ribs (1, 2, 11, 12)

The 1st and 2nd ribs are short and flattened (Fig. 3.15.6). The 11th and 12th ribs articulate posteriorly with only one vertebra.

Sternum

The sternum (Fig. 3.15.1) develops from four cartilages (sternebrae) that fuse during development. Failure to fuse may result in a persistent hole in the body or xiphoid process. The joint between the manubrium and the body is the **sternal angle** (angle of Louis). It is an important surface landmark for the 2nd costal cartilage (indicating vertebral level T4).

The sternum has three parts (Fig. 3.15.1):

- **manubrium:** the upper border is the jugular (suprasternal) notch at the level of T2; the clavicles articulate on each side and the arch of the aorta lies posteriorly
- **body:** lies between T5 and T9 with the heart lying posteriorly; the body is a convenient site to sample bone marrow (sternal tap)
- **xiphoid:** very variable in shape, it sometimes ossifies later in life.

Thoracic vertebrae are described on p. 28.

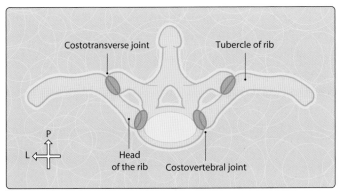

Fig. 3.15.4 Transverse section of the 5th thoracic vertebra and its articulations with the 5th ribs.

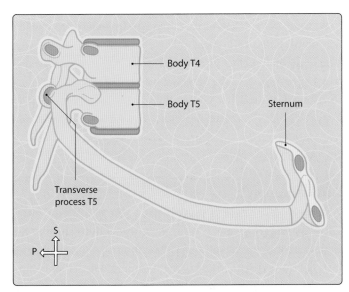

Fig. 3.15.5 Lateral view of the 5th rib and its posterior articulation with the 4th and 5th thoracic vertebrae and its anterior articulation with the sternum.

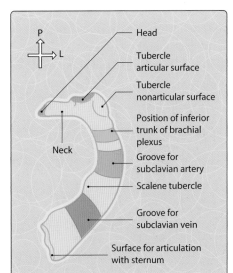

Fig. 3.15.6 View of the 1st rib from above.

CERVICAL RIBS

An extra pair of ribs can occur in the neck (cervical ribs). Cervical ribs may compress the inferior trunk of the brachial plexus leading to weakness and wasting of the intrinsic muscles of the hand and paraesthesia over the ulnar border of the forearm (dermatomes C8 and T1; p. 7).

16. Chest wall and intercostal spaces

Questions
- What types of nerve fibre are carried in the intercostal nerves?
- Which dermatome lies at the level of the umbilicus?
- Where is it safe to insert a chest drain?

Intercostal spaces

There are three layers of muscle in the body wall (Fig. 3.16.1). They form three thin sheets in the abdomen and, in the thorax, they fill the intercostal spaces from the inferior edge of the rib above to the superior border of the rib below. When they contract they lift the rib below towards the rib above.

- The **external intercostal** muscle fibres run downwards and medially (like your hands in your trouser pockets); they fill the most posterior and lateral parts of the space but are replaced by a membrane anteriorly. It is equivalent to the external oblique of the abdominal wall.
- The **internal intercostal** fibres run downwards and laterally filling the anterior and lateral parts of the space but are replaced by a membrane posteriorly; the **neurovascular bundle** lies in the costal groove between the second and third layers of muscle (from top the bundle consists of intercostal vein, artery and nerve (VAN)). It is equivalent to the internal oblique of the abdominal wall.
- The **innermost intercostal** muscle is an incomplete layer that is not important in breathing movements; it is

confusing because it is not named consistently. It is equivalent to the transversus abdominis of the abdominal wall.

Nerves

The lateral and anterior body wall is innervated by the ventral primary rami of thoracic spinal nerves (Fig. 3.16.2).

1. Each nerve emerges from the intervertebral foramen below its own numbered vertebra.
2. Each nerve divides into **dorsal and ventral rami**: dorsal rami supply the erector spinae muscles and skin of the back; ventral rami (intercostal nerves) supply the anterior two-thirds of the body wall (thorax and abdomen).
3. Each thoracic spinal nerve is connected to a sympathetic ganglion through the **white ramus communicans**; it carries preganglionic sympathetic fibres to the ganglion
4. The **grey ramus communicans** connects the sympathetic ganglion back to the spinal nerve and carries postganglionic sympathetic fibres.

Each nerve also
- gives a **collateral branch** at the angle of the rib, which carries mainly motor fibres
- gives **lateral cutaneous branches** in the mid-axillary line that supply the lateral skin of the thorax
- gives **motor branches** to the intercostal muscles
- gives **sensory branches** to the parietal pleura
- carries **sympathetic fibres** to the blood vessels, arrector pili muscles of hair follicles and sweat glands of the thoracic body wall (see p. 74)
- terminates as the **anterior cutaneous branch** supplying skin on the anterior thoracic wall.

The C_4 dermatome lies immediately above the sternal angle and just below it is T_2. The intervening dermatomes (C_5–T_1) are distributed around the upper limb. Skin over the xiphoid is supplied by T_7. Intercostal nerves T_8–T_{12} supply the muscles and skin of the anterior abdominal wall, with T_{10} lying at the level of the umbilicus (see p. 7).

Arterial supply

Anteriorly, each space is supplied by a pair of **anterior intercostal arteries** (Fig. 3.16.2) from the **internal thoracic artery**, a branch of the subclavian artery. The internal thoracic arteries pass inferiorly on either side of the sternum immediately behind the costal cartilages. The branches supply the anterior part of the intercostal spaces and the lateral half of the breast. The internal thoracic artery terminates by dividing into the **musculophrenic**

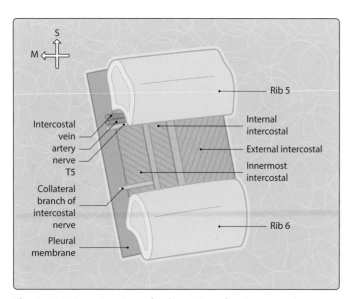

Fig. 3.16.1 Anterior view of a dissection of an intercostal space to show the intercostal muscles and neurovascular bundle.

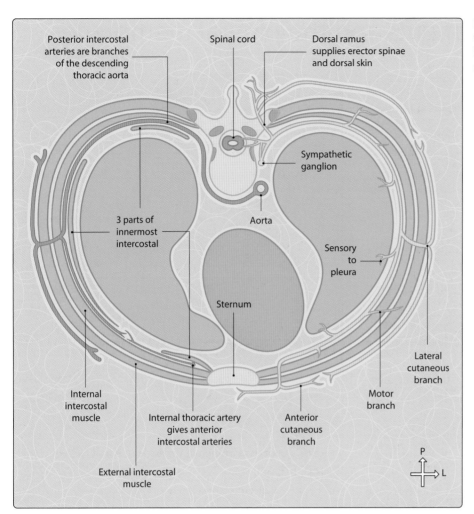

Fig. 3.16.2 Cross-section of the thoracic wall showing the arrangement of intercostal muscles and neurovascular structures.

Posterior intercostal arteries are branches of the descending thoracic aorta

Spinal cord

Dorsal ramus supplies erector spinae and dorsal skin

Sympathetic ganglion

3 parts of innermost intercostal

Aorta

Sensory to pleura

Sternum

Internal intercostal muscle

Internal thoracic artery gives anterior intercostal arteries

Anterior cutaneous branch

Motor branch

Lateral cutaneous branch

External intercostal muscle

P
L

artery, which supplies the diaphragm and inferior intercostal spaces, and the **superior epigastric artery**, which continues inferiorly to enter the rectus sheath, where it will anastomose with the inferior epigastric artery (p. 76).

Posteriorly the upper two intercostal spaces are supplied by the costocervical branch of the subclavian artery. The remaining spaces are supplied by direct branches of the descending thoracic aorta. These branches not only supply the intercostal space but also give important branches to the spinal cord in this region.

Venous drainage

Anteriorly, intercostal veins drain *via* the internal thoracic veins to the brachiocephalic veins (Fig. 3.16.1). The larger posterior veins drain into a network of interconnected venous channels lying on the vertebral bodies, known as the **azygos system** (p. 69). It not only drains the intercostal veins on each side of the body but also forms a connection between the inferior and superior venae cavae and with the vertebral venous plexus that drains the spinal cord and vertebrae. This anatomical connection explains how breast cancer can spread to the bone marrow cavity of thoracic vertebrae, where secondary tumours may develop.

 INSERTION OF A CHEST DRAIN

It may be necessary to insert a drain (thoracocentesis) to remove excess fluid or air from the pleural cavity. To avoid damage to major viscera or to the neurovascular bundle, the tube is inserted into the lower part of the intercostal space:
■ either in the 2nd intercostal space in the mid-clavicular line
■ or in the 4th or 5th space in the mid-axillary line.

17. Breathing movements and the pleural membranes

Questions
- How is the volume of the chest increased during breathing movements?
- What normally causes expiration?
- What are the surface markings of the pleurae and where do they extend beyond the thoracic cage?

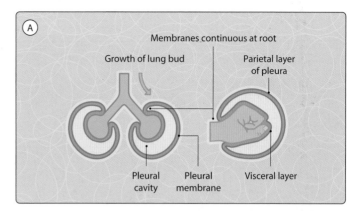

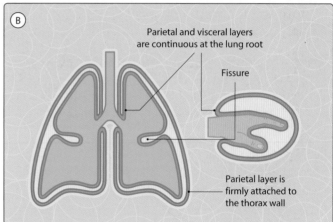

Fig. 3.17.1 Diagrammatic representations of the concept of invagination. (A) Pushing the hand into a balloon demonstrates the early development of the lung buds as they grow into the pleural cavities. (B) The open hand pushed into the balloon represents the later, more complex development of the lungs and pleura, showing that all the surfaces of the lungs are covered by the visceral pleura.

BREATHING MOVEMENTS

Inspiration: is brought about by movements that increase the volume of the thoracic cage.

- increase in the vertical diameter: the diaphragm contracts and flattens
- increase in the anteroposterior diameter: contraction of the intercostal muscles raises the upper ribs and lifts the sternum like a pump handle
- increase in the transverse diameter: contraction of the intercostal muscles raises the costal margin and lower ribs like a series of bucket handles.

In deep inspiration, additional muscles may help to increase the volume of the thorax (sternocleidomastoid, pectoralis major and latissimus dorsi).

Expiration is normally a passive process as muscles relax and the stretched elastic tissue of the inflated lungs and bronchial tree recoil (like a balloon deflating). Expiration becomes an active process in diseases such as emphysema where the elasticity of the lungs is impaired. Rapid, powerful contraction of the anterior abdominal muscles causes forced expiration (e.g. coughing).

PLEURAE

The mediastinum lies in the centre of the thorax and on either side are the lungs in their separate **pleural cavities**. The cavities are lined by the pleural membranes (simple squamous epithelium).

During development, the lungs grow into the pleural cavities and become covered by the epithelium that lines the cavity. The thoracic wall is lined by the **parietal pleura** and the covering of the lung is the **visceral pleura** (Fig. 3.17.1). Normally, only a thin film of lubricating fluid separates the two layers of pleura. The fluid acts like a thin film of water trapped between two sheets of glass, they can slide past one another but the surface tension between them does not allow them to be pulled apart. On inspiration, the chest wall and its lining parietal pleura move outwards, and a slight negative pressure between the pleurae ensures that the visceral pleura and lung are pulled out with the chest wall causing the lung to inflate.

The point at which the lung enters the pleural cavity is known as the **root** of the lung. This is the only region where the bronchi, blood vessels and nerves enter or leave the lung and here the parietal and visceral layers are not separate but are just one continuous layer. Different areas of the parietal pleura are named according to the structures they overlie (e.g. costal, diaphragmatic).

It is important to know the **surface markings** of the pleural cavities. The apex of the pleural cavity lies 2.5 cm above the medial end of the clavicle. Right and left pleurae are adjacent in the midline at the 2nd costal cartilage. There is a small cardiac notch on the left between the 4th and 6th costal cartilages. In the midclavicular line, the pleurae lie at the level of the 8th rib, in the midaxillary line at the 10th rib and in the midscapular line at the level of the 12th rib. Remember that they extend beyond

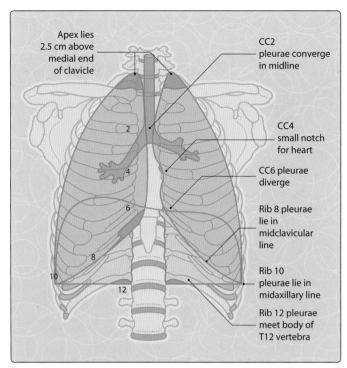

Fig. 3.17.2 Anterior view of the thoracic cage showing the surface markings for the pleura and the position of the trachea and main bronchi. Areas coloured dark pink show the sites where the pleural cavities project beyond the thoracic cage. CC, costal cartilage.

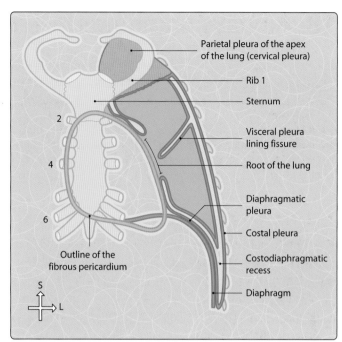

Fig. 3.17.4 Coronal section of the thorax showing the position of the costodiaphragmatic recess.

the bony thoracic cage, where they become vulnerable to puncture injuries (Figs 3.17.2–3.17.4)

- in the root of the neck they rise 2.5 cm above the clavicle
- below the right costal margin (closely related to the liver)
- below the 12th rib close to the vertebral column on each side (closely related to the kidneys).

Pleura recesses

In quiet inspiration, the lungs do not completely fill the pleural cavities. The resulting spaces are known as the costomediastinal and costodiaphragmatic pleural recesses (Figs 3.17.3 and 3.17.4).

 PNEUMOTHORAX

Normally, the lungs remain partially inflated even after expiration. If air enters the pleural space, the surface tension between the pleural membranes is lost, the lung completely deflates and collapses away from the wall preventing normal inflation of the lung (pneumothorax). It can be caused by a stabbing injury where atmospheric air enters the space. It can also occur spontaneously if a weakness in the visceral pleura allows air from the lung to escape into the space. Pneumothorax is treated by the insertion of a chest drain (p. 57). Because the pleural cavities are separate, collapse of one lung will not cause collapse of the other.

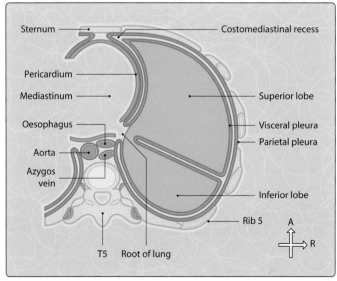

Fig. 3.17.3 Cross-section of the thorax at the level of T5 showing the position of the pleurae, lungs and mediastinum.

18. Airways and lungs

Questions
- If you choke on a peanut where is it most likely to be found?
- If a patient is lying down, in which lobes of the lungs is fluid likely to accumulate?
- Why is it important to understand the lymphatic drainage of the lungs?

Trachea and bronchi

The trachea begins below the cricoid cartilage of the larynx at C_6 where it is closely related to the thyroid gland and oesophagus (p. 156). The C-shaped rings of cartilage that keep the airway open can be felt in the midline of the neck between the sterno-clavicular joints. The branching pattern of the bronchial tree is constant and allows prediction of the position at which foreign bodies can lodge, where fluid will collect and how disease will spread. The divisions occur as follows.

- The **trachea** divides behind the sternal angle.
- The two **main** (principal) **bronchi** enter the hilum of the lung with the pulmonary vessels; the right main bronchus is shorter, wider and more vertical than the left (for this reason, if you choke on a peanut it is likely to lodge in the right lung) (Fig. 3.17.2, p. 59).
- There are five **lobar bronchi**, three on the right and two on the left.
- The **segmental bronchi,** ten on the right and nine on the left, supply wedge-shaped **bronchopulmonary segments.** The segments lie with their base on the visceral pleura and apex pointing to the root of the lung. Each segment has its own bronchus, artery, vein and lymphatics and is divided from adjacent segments by connective tissue. Disease may be confined to an individual segment. The apical and lower segments of the posterior lobes are the sites where fluid is likely to accumulate in patients lying on their backs and this is the commonest site of infections in bedridden patients (see Fig. 3.18.1 and Table 3.18.1).
- Subsequent divisions form increasingly narrower diameter airways (**bronchioles**) terminating in millions of microscopic air sacs, the **alveoli.**

Lungs

The lungs are cone shaped with an apex that rises up into the root of the neck and a concave base that lies over the diaphragm (Fig. 3.18.2). Because the heart lies mainly on the left side, the right lung is slightly larger than the left and is divided into three lobes, upper, middle and lower, by oblique and horizontal fissures. The left lung is deeply indented by the heart and has only an oblique fissure to separate upper and lower lobes (Fig. 3.18.2).

Blood supply

The pulmonary circulation consists of the:

- **pulmonary arteries**, which bring venous blood from the right ventricle; they divide extensively to present an enormous capillary surface in the walls of the alveoli to allow efficient gaseous exchange

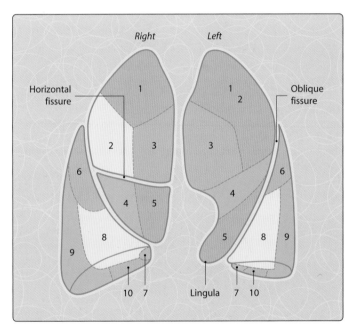

Fig. 3.18.1 Anterior view of the bronchopulmonary segments (numbers refer to Table 3.18.1).

Table 3.18.1 BRONCHOPULMONARY SEGMENTS (see Fig. 3.18.1)

Segment	Right lung	Left lung
Superior lobe		
1	Apical	Apicoposterior
2	Posterior	Apicoposterior
3	Anterior	Anterior
Middle lobe		
4	Lateral	Superior lingular
5	Medial	Inferior lingular
Inferior lobe		
6	Apical basal	Apical basal
7	Anterior basal	Anterior basal
8	Medial basal	Medial basal
9	Lateral basal	Lateral basal
10	Posterior basal	Posterior basal

- **pulmonary veins**, which carry oxygenated blood back to the left atrium for distribution to the systemic circulation
- **bronchial arteries**, which are direct branches of the aorta that supply the walls of the airways.

Lymphatic drainage

Lymph drains from the lung to the **bronchopulmonary nodes** at the hilum (sometimes called the hilar nodes; Fig. 3.18.3). These drain to a large group of **tracheobronchial nodes** lying at the bifurcation of the trachea. Lymph is carried from this important group of nodes to the bronchomediastinal lymph trunks, which usually empty directly into the great veins.

Nerve supply

The lungs are innervated by the **pulmonary plexus,** consisting of direct branches from the sympathetic trunk and pulmonary branches of the vagus nerve. Sympathetic stimulation dilates the bronchioles. Asthma is caused by contraction of smooth muscle, which narrows the bronchioles. Treatment involves inhalation of drugs that mimic sympathetic stimulation.

Surface markings

The landmarks on the lung are the same as for the pleurae but the cardiac notch is larger and the inferior borders are two inter-costal spaces shorter; the difference between the two is the costodiaphragmatic recess (Fig. 3.18.3).

The apex lies 2.5 cm above the clavicle. The lungs and pleurae meet in the midline at the level of the 2nd costal cartilages. The cardiac notch lies between the 4th and 6th costal cartilages on the left. The inferior border of the lungs lies at the level of the 6th rib in the midclavicular line, the 8th rib in the midaxillary line and 10th rib with midscapular line.

 LUNG CANCER

Bronchial carcinoma is the commonest cancer in men in the UK. It occurs most frequently in the mucous membrane lining the major bronchi and spreads to the hilar and tracheobronchial nodes at an early stage. If the tracheobronchial nodes become enlarged, they may distort the internal anatomy of the trachea at its bifurcation (the carina), which can be observed using a bronchoscope.

Fig. 3.18.2 Anterior view of the thoracic cage showing the surface markings for the lobes of the lungs.

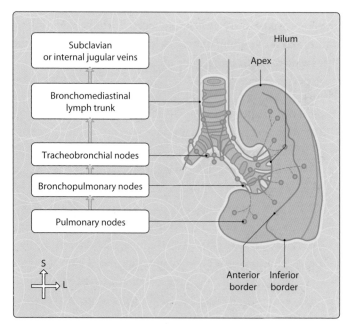

Fig. 3.18.3 Diagrammatic representation of the lymphatic drainage of the left lung.

19. Pericardium and heart: the middle mediastinum

Questions
- Which chambers of the heart make up the borders of the cardiac shadow in a radiograph of the chest?
- Which chamber of the heart is closely related to the oesophagus?
- What events cause the first and second heart sounds?

The heart, surrounded by the **fibrous pericardium,** lies immediately behind the body of the sternum (T5–T9). The pericardium and its contents are known as the middle **mediastinum** (p. 66).

Pericardium

The fibrous pericardium is attached superiorly to the roots of the great vessels and inferiorly to the central tendon of the diaphragm (Fig. 3.22.1, p. 68). Within this fibrous sac, the heart is covered by two layers of **serous pericardium**. The **parietal layer** is firmly attached to the inside surface of the fibrous pericardium and the **visceral pericardium** covers the surfaces of the heart. Between the two serous layers is a thin film of fluid, which allows the heart to beat in a friction-free environment. The pericardium is supplied by the **phrenic nerves** (p. 70).

Heart

The heart is divided into four chambers (Figs 3.19.1–3.19.3).

The **right** and **left atria** have thin muscular walls; they contract simultaneously filling the ventricles (diastole). The right atrium receives blood from the inferior and superior venae cavae and the coronary sinus, the left atrium from the pulmonary veins. They are separated by the **interatrial septum,** which may fail to develop normally leading to atrial septal defect.

The **right** and **left ventricles** have thick muscular walls; they contract simultaneously (systole) pumping blood away from the heart. Contraction of the right ventricle forces blood into the pulmonary trunk and the lungs at a diastolic pressure of 35 mmHg. The more powerful left ventricle pumps blood into the aorta and the systemic circulation at a systolic pressure of 120 mmHg. The interventricular septum has a complex developmental origin and may be defective, leading to a serious condition known as ventricular septal defect.

Two sets of **valves** ensure the one-way flow of blood through the heart (Fig. 3.19.4). **Atrioventricular valves** (right, tricuspid; left, bicuspid/mitral) prevent backflow of blood into the atria during systole. The pressure of the ventricular contraction causes the cusps of the valves to fill with blood and to close making the first heart sound (LUB). The papillary muscles and the chordae

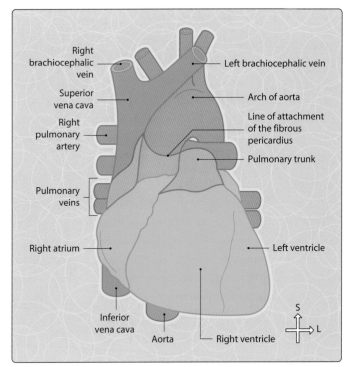

Fig. 3.19.1 Anterior view showing the sternocostal surface of the heart and great vessels.

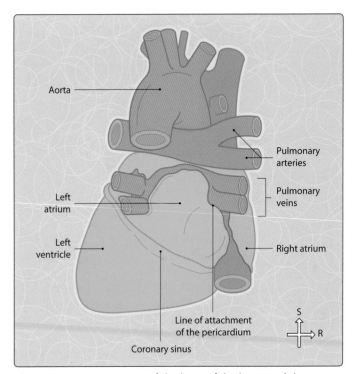

Fig. 3.19.2 Posterior view of the base of the heart and the great vessels.

tendineae attached to the edges of the cusps prevent the cusps from being forced into the atrium during ventricular contraction or systole. The **pulmonary** and **aortic valves** prevent backflow into the ventricles during diastole. Each has three semilunar cusps that fill with blood, closing the valves and causing the second heart sound (DUB).

Borders of the heart

Examine Fig. 3.19.3 carefully; you need to know which chambers form the **borders** of the heart to interpret chest radiographs:

- superior border: the great vessels; 2nd to 3rd costal cartilages
- right border: right atrium; 3rd to 5th right costal cartilages
- inferior border: right ventricle; 5th right costal cartilage to apex beat in 5th intercostal space
- left border; left ventricle and auricle of left atrium; apex beat to 2nd left costal cartilage.

Surfaces of the heart

Because the human chest is flattened, the heart is partly rotated to the left (Fig. 3.19.5).

- **anterior/sternocostal surface**: right atrium and ventricle, thin strip of left ventricle and atrium
- **inferior/diaphragmatic surface**: right and left ventricles lie on the diaphragm
- **posterior/base**: left atrium lies immediately anterior to the oesophagus.

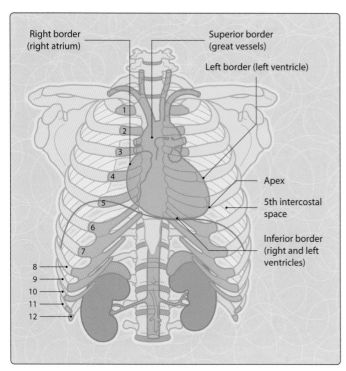

Fig. 3.19.3 Anterior view of the thorax showing the surface markings of the heart.

Right border (right atrium)
Superior border (great vessels)
Left border (left ventricle)
1
2
3
4
Apex
5
5th intercostal space
6
7
Inferior border (right and left ventricles)
8
9
10
11
12

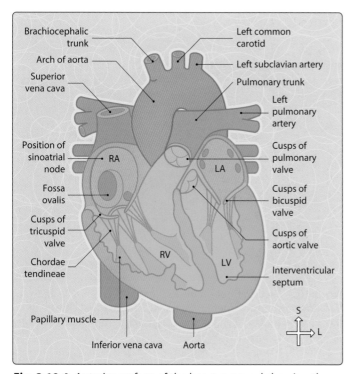

Fig. 3.19.4 Anterior surface of the heart removed showing the valves and other major internal structures.

Brachiocephalic trunk
Arch of aorta
Superior vena cava
Position of sinoatrial node
RA
Fossa ovalis
Cusps of tricuspid valve
Chordae tendineae
RV
LV
Papillary muscle
Inferior vena cava
Aorta
Left common carotid
Left subclavian artery
Pulmonary trunk
Left pulmonary artery
Cusps of pulmonary valve
LA
Cusps of bicuspid valve
Cusps of aortic valve
Interventricular septum
S
L

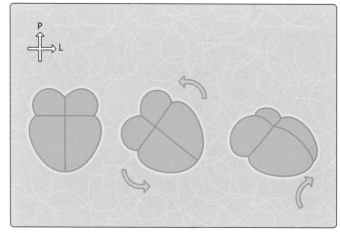

Fig. 3.19.5 Rotation of the human heart.

P
L
S
L

 CARDIAC TAMPONADE

The fibrous pericardium is tough and inelastic. If thoracic trauma causes bleeding into the pericardium from the coronary arteries, the heart becomes increasingly constricted and cannot fill normally (cardiac tamponade). It is a potentially fatal emergency.

20. Coronary arteries and innervation of the heart

Questions
- Which chambers of the heart are supplied by the left coronary artery?
- Which important component of the conducting system lies in the interventricular septum?
- What is myocardial infarction?

On average, the heart contracts 72 times every minute. The myocardium needs a rich blood supply to maintain this level of activity, which means its own arterial supply.

Coronary arteries

The right and left coronary arteries (RCA and LCA) arise from the **aortic sinuses** just above the cusps of the aortic valve (Fig. 3.20.1). When the aortic valve closes during diastole, the sinuses fill with blood and blood flows into the coronary arteries (Figs 3.20.2 and 3.20.3). They lie on the external surface of the heart, embedded in fatty tissue in the atrioventricular (AV) and interventricular grooves (Fig. 3.20.4).

The RCA opens from the anterior aortic sinus and passes inferiorly in the AV groove, giving a marginal branch along the inferior border. Turning under the heart onto the diaphragmatic

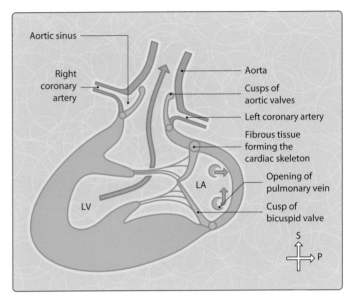

Fig. 3.20.2 Section through the left atrium, left ventricle and aortic valve showing closure of the mitral valve and opening of the aortic valve during systole.

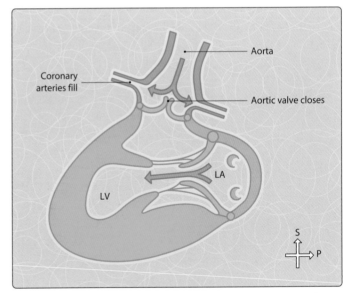

Fig. 3.20.3 Section through the left atrium, left ventricle and aortic valve showing opening of the mitral valve and closure of the aortic valve and filling of the coronary arteries during diastole.

surface, it gives a posterior interventricular branch before it terminates by anastomosing with the LCA. It supplies both atria and the posterior part of the interventricular septum and both ventricles. In most people it supplies the sinuatrial node.

The LCA arises from the left posterior aortic sinus. As the artery enters the AV groove, it divides into two branches. The **anterior** (or **descending**) **interventricular branch** passes

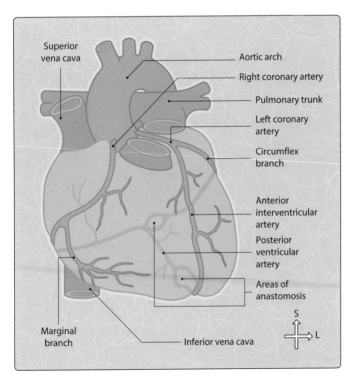

Fig. 3.20.1 Anterior view of the sternocostal surface of the heart showing the coronary arteries.

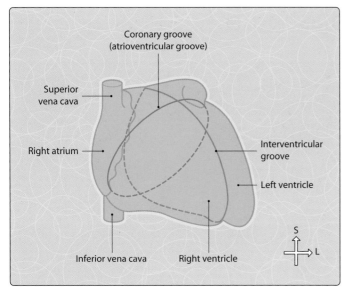

Fig. 3.20.4 Anterior view of the heart showing the position of the grooves between the chambers.

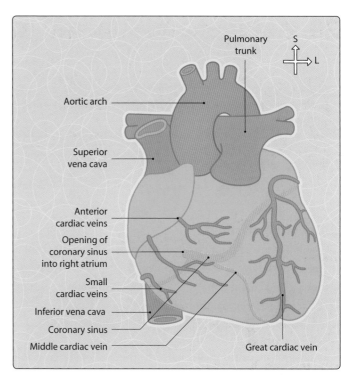

Fig. 3.20.5 Anterior view of the sternocostal surface of the heart to show the major veins.

inferiorly in the interventricular groove and turns under the heart to anastomose with the interventricular branch of the RCA on the diaphragmatic surface. The **circumflex branch** passes posteriorly in the AV groove to anastomose with the RCA. The LCA supplies both atria, the anterior part of the interventricular septum and both ventricles.

Cardiac veins

The cardiac veins accompany the coronary arteries and drain to the coronary sinus, which empties into the right atrium (Fig. 3.20.5).

Conducting system

Myocardial cells contract spontaneously without nervous stimulation and different regions of the heart contract at different rates (ventricles beat more slowly than atria). The region that contracts most rapidly will impose its rate on the rest of the heart. The **sinuatrial node** has the fastest inherent rate and is, therefore, the **pacemaker** (Fig. 3.19.4, p. 63). The rate of heart beat is modulated by the cardiac plexus consisting of:

- **cardiac branches** of the **vagus nerve**, which slow the rate (bradycardia; p. 72)
- **sympathetic branches** from the cervical and thoracic sympathetic ganglia increase rate and force of contraction (tachycardia; p. 74).

The contraction initiated by the sinuatrial node spreads across the atrial walls but is prevented from crossing directly into the ventricles by the fibrous skeleton that reinforces the base of the AV valves (Fig. 3.20.2). The impulse is carried from the AV node via the AV bundle. The bundle lies in the interventricular septum, where it divides to form the **bundles of His**. The rate of conduction of the impulse in the bundles delays systole until the ventricles are filled following diastole. The blood supply of the bundles is mainly derived from the anterior interventricular branch of the LCA. It is this branch that is most commonly affected by atherosclerosis and, therefore, most commonly replaced in coronary artery bypass surgery.

 HEART ATTACK

Although there are anastomoses between the RCA and LCA, the vessels are minute (arterioles), which makes the coronary arteries **functional end arteries**. If a coronary artery is blocked suddenly by thrombus, the myocardium is deprived of blood because the anastomoses cannot support a collateral circulation and a heart attack (myocardial infarction) will occur.

In ischaemic heart disease, atheroma causes narrowing of the coronary arteries over a period of time and patients complain of increasing chest pain (angina). Angina may be controlled pharmacologically or surgically by coronary artery bypass graft.

21. Anterior and superior mediastinum

Questions
- What is the arrangement of the neurovascular structures that lie on the first rib?
- Which bony landmark indicates the bifurcation of the trachea?
- Which part of the aorta lies behind the manubrium?

Anterior mediastinum

The anterior mediastinum is a narrow space immediately behind the body of the sternum (Figs 3.21.1 and 3.21.2). It is filled by the thymus gland in children but this atrophies in adults, leaving only fat and the internal thoracic arteries.

Superior mediastinum

The superior mediastinum includes the thoracic inlet (Fig. 3.21.1) and is continuous with the root of neck (p. 155). It is a complex region. It may help you to recall:

- **arrangement of structures on the first rib**: most anterior is the subclavian vein, behind it is the subclavian artery, the brachial plexus lies posterior to the artery but does not enter the thorax (Fig. 3.66.2; p. 156); the relationship between veins and arteries is maintained in the thorax
- **asymmetry in the thorax** arises because veins drain to the right side of the heart and arteries arise from the left; structures on the right are, therefore, related to *veins and the right atrium* and on the left to *arteries and the left ventricle.*

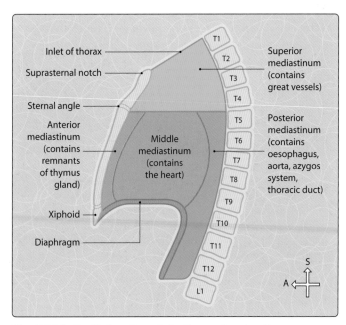

Fig. 3.21.1 Sagittal section of the thorax showing the subdivisions of the mediastinum.

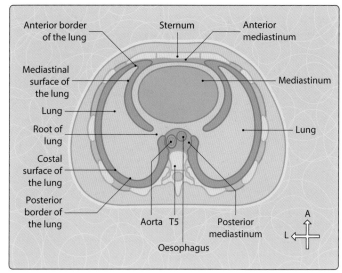

Fig. 3.21.2 Cross section of the thorax at T5 showing the position of the lungs and mediastinum.

From anterior to posterior the major structures are the venous plane, arterial plane, trachea, oesophagus.

Venous plane

Immediately behind the manubrium lie the great veins (Fig. 3.21.3). They are related to four consecutive bony landmarks; they are **posterior** to the:

- **right sternoclavicular joint:** the subclavian and internal jugular veins join to form the brachiocephalic veins; the **thoracic duct** drains into the venous system at the junction of the left brachiocephalic and jugular veins
- **first right costal cartilage:** the left brachiocephalic vein crosses the midline to join the right brachiocephalic vein forming the superior vena cava (SVC)
- **second right costal cartilage:** SVC joined posteriorly by the azygos vein
- **third right costal cartilage:** SVC enters the right atrium.

Arterial plane

At its origin, the **aortic valve** lies posterior to the pulmonary trunk. As the ascending aorta and pulmonary trunk spiral around each other, the aorta comes to lie on the right of the pulmonary trunk (Fig. 3.21.3). The **coronary arteries** arise from the aortic sinuses of the ascending aorta (p. 64).

The **arch of the aorta** lies behind the manubrium. It begins at the level of the sternal angle (T4). It passes upwards, backwards and to the left over the left main bronchus. It ends posteriorly opposite T4 and continues as the descending thoracic aorta. There are three branches from the arch:

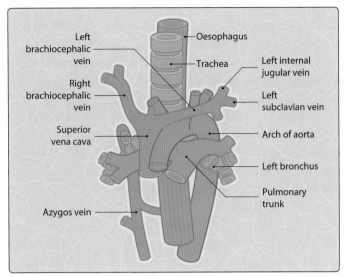

Fig. 3.21.3 The relations of the great vessels, trachea and oesophagus.

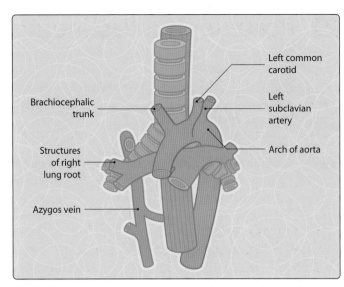

Fig. 3.21.4 The relations of the great vessels, trachea and oesophagus after removal of the major veins.

- **brachiocephalic trunk** arises in the midline and passes upwards to the right of the trachea; behind the sternoclavicular joint it divides to form the **right subclavian** and **right common carotid arteries**
- **left common carotid** passes to the left of the trachea
- **left subclavian** passes to the left of the trachea and crosses the 1st rib
- the common carotid arteries pass superiorly to supply the head and neck (p. 138).

The subclavian arteries supply the upper limbs by continuing as the axillary arteries. **The pulmonary trunk** (Figs 3.21.4 and 3.21.5) spirals to the left of the aorta. It divides under the arch of the aorta into the right and left pulmonary arteries.

Trachea and oesophagus

The bifurcation of the trachea (Fig. 3.21.6) and its associated tracheobronchial lymph nodes lie at the level of the sternal angle. The oesophagus begins in the neck at C6, posterior to the trachea in the midline of the neck and thoracic inlet (Fig. 3.21.6).

 CENTRAL LINES

The right brachiocephalic vein lies in almost a straight line from its formation behind the sternoclavicular joint to the superior vena cava and right atrium. The subclavian artery lies behind the vein, curving over the apex of the lung. A minor error in inserting a central line into the vein could result in a pneumothorax!

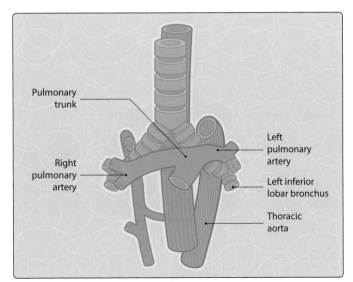

Fig. 3.21.5 The relations of the pulmonary arteries, trachea and oesophagus after removal of the major veins and the aortic arch.

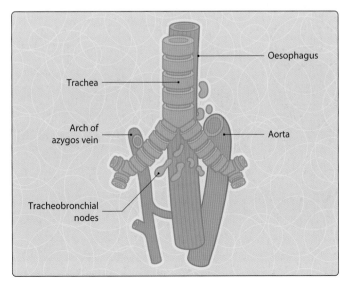

Fig. 3.21.6 The relations of the trachea, oesophagus, azygos vein and tracheobronchial lymph nodes.

22. Posterior mediastinum

Questions
- Which three structures indent the oesophagus, as seen in a normal barium swallow?
- Which structures pass through the aortic hiatus in the diaphragm?
- Where does the thoracic duct drain into the venous system?

The posterior mediastinum (p. 66) is a narrow space posterior to the pericardium and diaphragm and anterior to the bodies of the thoracic vertebrae T5–T12. It contains the oesophagus, thoracic aorta, azygos and hemiazygos veins and thoracic duct (Figs 3.22.1 and 3.22.2).

Oesophagus
Since the oesophagus connects the pharynx to the stomach on the *left* of the abdomen, it comes to lie to the *left* of the midline. It is slightly compressed as it passes:
- posterior to the *left* bronchus
- posterior to the *left* atrium
- forwards and pierces the diaphragm at T10 to the *left* of the central tendon to enter the stomach.

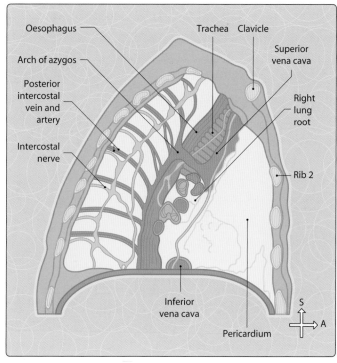

Fig. 3.22.2 View of the mediastinum from the right with the lung and pleura removed.

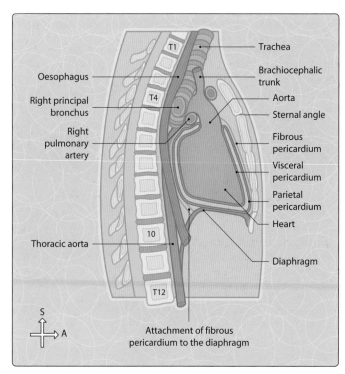

Fig. 3.22.1 Sagittal section of the thorax in the midline viewed from the right, showing the structures in the posterior mediastinum.

The blood supply and venous drainage of the oesophagus is complex:
- the **upper third** is supplied by the inferior thyroid artery and drains to the equivalent veins
- the **middle third** is supplied directly from the aorta and drains to the azygos system
- the **lower third** is supplied by the left gastric artery and drains to left gastric veins and the hepatic portal system; this is a site of **portosystemic anastomosis** (p. 85).

Thoracic aorta
The **descending thoracic aorta** is the continuation of the aortic arch at the level of T4 (Figs 3.22.1 and 3.22.3). It lies on the left side of the posterior mediastinum in contact with the vertebral bodies. It approaches the midline and passes through the **aortic hiatus** of the diaphragm at the level of T12 with the thoracic duct and the azygos vein. It continues as the abdominal aorta. Its branches are:
- segmental branches to each intercostal space except the first two, which are supplied from a branch of the subclavian artery
- three bronchial arteries to the tissue of the lungs
- oesophageal branches.

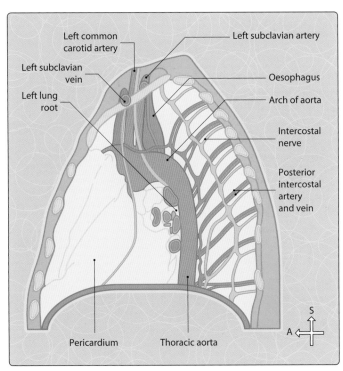

Fig. 3.22.3 View of the mediastinum from the left with the lung and pleura removed.

Azygos system

The veins of the azygos system are very variable. Segmental veins of the posterior abdominal wall (lumbar veins) and posterior wall of the thorax (posterior intercostal veins) drain to the azygos vein on the right and to the hemiazygos on the left (Figs 3.22.2 and 3.22.4).

■ the **azygos vein** has connections with the inferior vena cava (IVC), passes through the diaphragm with the aorta and empties into the SVC; the terminal part of the azygos arches over the right lung root to empty into the SVC

■ the **hemiazygos vein** arises from the left renal vein and drains to the azygos across the midline at about T8.

Thoracic duct

The thoracic duct is the main lymphatic channel of the body (p. 39). It receives lymph from the entire body except the right side of the head and neck, right upper limb and right side of the thorax. It begins in the abdomen just below the diaphragm from the cysterna chyli and passes through the aortic hiatus with the aorta and azygos vein. In the region of T4, it crosses to the left and passing through the thoracic inlet drains into the venous

system at the junction of the left brachiocephalic and jugular veins. Abdominal cancer can spread via the thoracic duct to the left supraclavicular nodes.

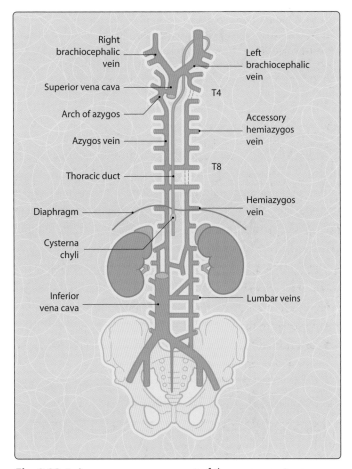

Fig. 3.22.4 A common arrangement of the azygos system showing the position of the thoracic duct.

SPREAD OF BREAST CANCER VIA THE AZYGOS VEINS

Tumours of the breast may metastasize to bodies of the thoracic vertebrae. Malignant cells can be carried via posterior intercostal veins to the azygos system. The azygos veins have no valves and receive tributaries from the vertebral venous plexus, which drains the spinal cord and bone marrow cavity of the thoracic vertebrae. Tumour cells may be carried into the marrow cavity, allowing the development of a secondary tumour. This is an example of haematogenic spread of cancer.

23. The diaphragm and phrenic nerves

Questions
- At which vertebral levels do the inferior vena cava, oesophagus and aorta pass through the diaphragm?
- At what level does the central tendon of the diaphragm lie after expiration? How does this relate to the normal position of the apex beat?
- To which dermatome is irritation of the diaphragm referred?

Diaphragm

The diaphragm separates the thorax from the abdomen and is the chief muscle of inspiration (Figs 3.23.1–3.23.4; see p. 58). It curves upwards into right and left domes; the right is higher than the left. The muscular fibres of the diaphragm arise from the xiphoid process anteriorly, costal cartilages 7–12 laterally and posteriorly from lumbar vertebrae by two crura and the arcuate ligaments (Fig. 3.23.1). They insert into a central tendon that lies at the level of the 5th rib during expiration; however, remember that the level varies with the phase of respiration and the position of the body. The central tendon is fused with the fibrous

pericardium. The embryological origins of the diaphragm are complex and defects may arise during development.

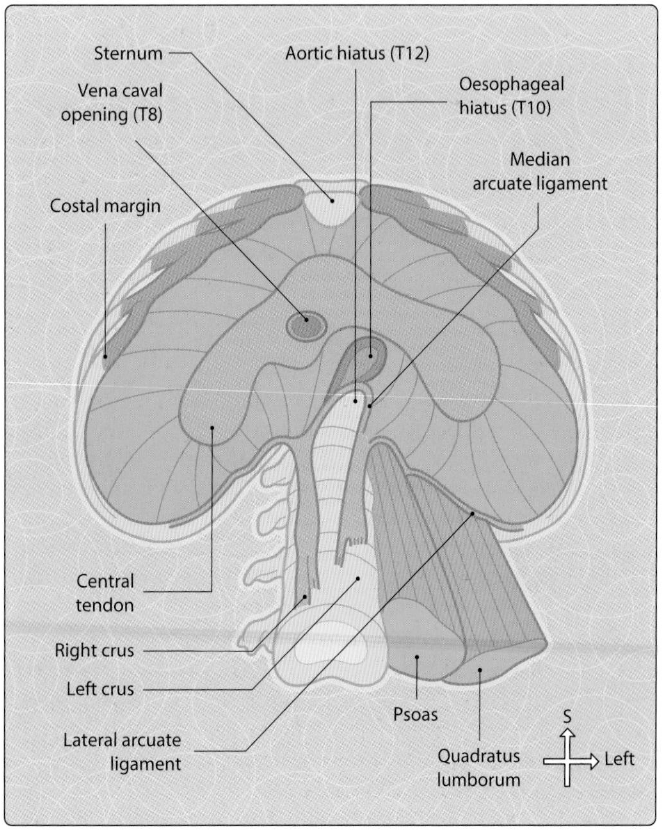

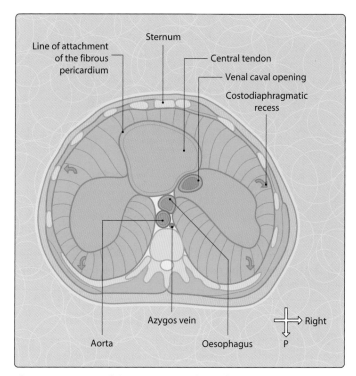

Fig. 3.23.2 View of the superior surface of the diaphragm from the thorax looking down.

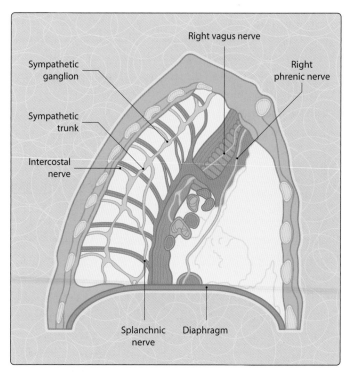

Fig. 3.23.3 View of the mediastinum from the right with the lung and pleura removed.

Fig. 3.23.1 View of the inferior surface of the diaphragm from the abdomen looking upwards.

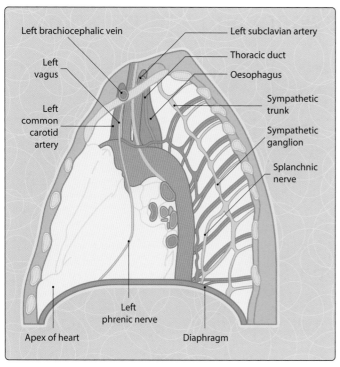

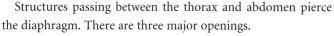

Fig. 3.23.4 View of the mediastinum from the left with the lung and pleura removed.

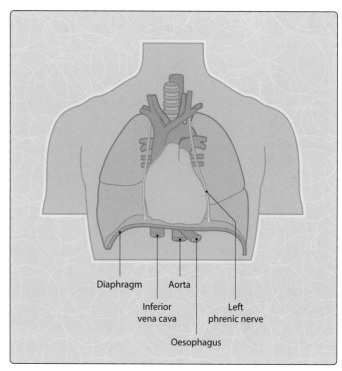

Fig. 3.23.5 Anterior view showing the position of the phrenic nerves.

Structures passing between the thorax and abdomen pierce the diaphragm. There are three major openings.

1. **Aortic hiatus** at **T12** lies behind the diaphragm for the thoracic aorta, thoracic duct and azygos vein.

2. **Oesophageal opening** at **T10** lies to the left of the midline in the muscular part of the diaphragm. Muscle fibres of the right crus loop around the oesophagus and act like a sphincter, constricting the oesophagus as the diaphragm contracts. The anterior and posterior vagal trunks lie on the oesophagus together with the oesophageal branches of the left gastric vessels.

3. **Caval opening** at **T8** lies in the central tendon for the IVC accompanied by the right phrenic nerve. The wall of the IVC is fused to the central tendon so that when the muscular part of the diaphragm contracts, the IVC dilates and the increased intra-abdominal pressure forces blood into the right atrium.

Phrenic nerves

The muscular periphery of the diaphragm develops from the innermost layer of the body wall muscle in the cervical region of the embryo. As the diaphragm shifts to its final thoracic position, the cervical nerves that were originally 'assigned' to it are retained. The phrenic nerves, therefore, arise from the ventral rami of C_3, C_4, C_5 (mainly C_4). They are branches of the cervical plexus (p. 155) and provide the *only* motor supply to the diaphragm (Fig. 3.23.5). They also give a sensory supply to the

central tendon of the diaphragm, pericardium and diaphragmatic pleura and peritoneum.

From the neck the phrenic nerves pass through the thoracic inlet between the venous and arterial planes.

The **right phrenic** nerve (Figs 3.23.3 and 3.23.5) lies on the SVC and the pericardium of the right atrium. It passes through the central tendon of the diaphragm with the IVC at T8 (i.e. lies on veins).

The **left phrenic** nerve (Figs 3.23.4 and 3.23.5) lies between the left common carotid and left subclavian arteries. It crosses the arch of the aorta and the left ventricle (i.e. lies on arteries). It pierces the diaphragm near the apex of the heart.

The nerves spread out on the undersurface of the diaphragm. Irritation of the diaphragmatic pleura or diaphragmatic peritoneum may be referred to the C4 dermatome, causing pain over the shoulder.

CERVICAL FRACTURES AND THE PHRENIC NERVE

Spinal fractures that damage the cervical segments of the spinal cord may seriously affect the ability to breathe. Fracture of a cervical vertebra that causes damage to the spinal cord *above* the level of C4 will result in the loss of all breathing movements because the phrenic and all the intercostal nerves will be affected. Damage below C4 will affect the intercostal nerves but not the phrenic nerves and so breathing is still possible.

24. Parasympathetic nervous system and vagus nerves

Questions
- Which division of the autonomic system conserves energy and promotes relaxation?
- Which cranial nerves carry parasympathetic nerve fibres?
- In general, where do parasympathetic ganglia lie, close to the spinal cord or close to the organ they supply?

Autonomic nervous system

We have no voluntary control over our heart rate, temperature regulation or the secretion of saliva. These are examples of body functions that are controlled by the autonomic nervous system. The autonomic nervous system consists of the parasympathetic and sympathetic divisions (see Fig. 1.2, p. 6). Characteristically, autonomic nerves consist of two-neurone chains. The cell body of the first (preganglionic) neurone lies in the CNS and the cell body of the second (postganglionic) neurone lies in a ganglion outside the CNS (Fig. 3.24.1).

- activation of the sympathetic system *consumes* energy for a 'fight or flight response': pale skin, cold sweat, dilated pupils, rapid breathing and pounding heart
- the sympathetic system also controls 'on-going' activities such as temperature regulation (constriction of peripheral blood vessels, sweating, contraction of arrector pili muscles, which make 'goose bumps' or your hair stand on end) and dilation of the pupil; these responses involve the whole body
- activation of the parasympathetic system *conserves* energy by promoting a 'rest and digest response', e.g. it reduces breathing and heart rate, increases gastrointestinal secretory activity, stimulates peristalsis and the secretion of saliva and tears.

Parasympathetic nervous system

Preganglionic parasympathetic neurones are found either in the brainstem or in the sacral part of the spinal cord (see Fig. 3.24.2). Their axons are carried in **cranial nerves (CN) III, VII, IX** and **X** (p. 136) and the **sacral spinal nerves S_2, S_3, S_4**. They synapse with postganglionic parasympathetic neurones in **parasympathetic ganglia**, which are situated close to their site of action, e.g. in the cardiac or pulmonary plexuses (Fig. 3.24.1).

Parasympathetic nerves supply:
- smooth muscle of the thoracic, abdominal and pelvic viscera
- smooth muscle of the eye, e.g. sphincter pupillae, ciliary muscles
- glands, secretomotor to, for example, salivary, lacrimal, gastric glands.

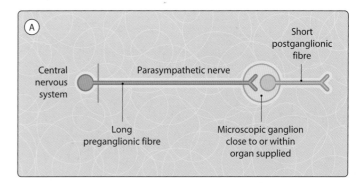

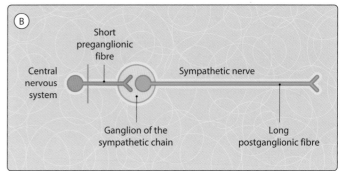

Fig. 3.24.1 Arrangement of the neurones of the autonomic system. (A) Parasympathetic; (B) sympathetic.

Note that there is *no* parasympathetic supply to blood vessels, the skin or limbs.

Vagus nerves

The vagus nerve is the 10th cranial nerve (CN X, Fig. 3.24.2). It carries preganglionic parasympathetic nerve fibres to thoracic and abdominal viscera as far as the left colic flexure.

In the neck, the vagus nerve lies in the carotid sheath between the common carotid artery and the internal jugular vein. The vagus nerves enter the thorax posterior to the brachiocephalic veins and anterior to the subclavian arteries.

The **right vagus** gives the **recurrent laryngeal branch,** which hooks under the right subclavian artery and passes upwards in the groove between the trachea and the oesophagus. It supplies the internal mucosa and intrinsic muscles of the larynx. The right vagus continues inferiorly on the right side of the trachea, passing behind the right lung root where it divides and contributes to the pulmonary, cardiac and oesophageal autonomic plexuses. The preganglionic neurones synapse in parasympathetic ganglia in the wall of the organ they supply and the postganglionic neurones innervate smooth muscle and glands.

The **left vagus** passes close to the origin of the common carotid artery and crosses the arch of the aorta, posterior to the phrenic nerve. It gives the left **recurrent laryngeal branch,**

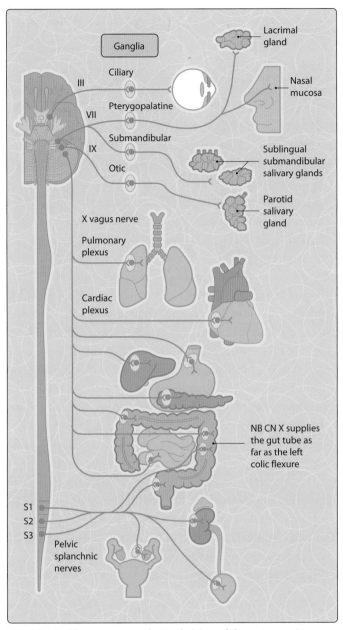

Ganglia

Ciliary

III

VII — Pterygopalatine

IX — Submandibular

Otic

X vagus nerve

Pulmonary plexus

Cardiac plexus

S1
S2
S3

Pelvic splanchnic nerves

Lacrimal gland

Nasal mucosa

Sublingual submandibular salivary glands

Parotid salivary gland

NB CN X supplies the gut tube as far as the left colic flexure

Fig. 3.24.2 The parasympathetic division of the autonomic nervous system.

which passes under the arch of the aorta and upwards to supply the larynx. The left vagus divides and mingles with the branches of the right vagus to form the cardiac, pulmonary and oesophageal plexuses.

The nerves are reconstituted on the surface of the oesophagus as the **anterior** and **posterior vagal trunks**. They pass through the diaphragm with the oesophagus at the level of T10.

The vagus nerves continue into the abdomen, branching to supply all the abdominal viscera as far as the left colic flexure (*vagus* means wandering). Parasympathetic innervation distally is derived from the pelvic splanchnic nerves.

LUNG CANCER AND THE RECURRENT LARYNGEAL NERVES

Bronchial carcinoma spreads quickly to the hilar and tracheo-bronchial nodes. The left recurrent laryngeal nerve is closely related to these nodes as it passes under the arch of the aorta. The left recurrent laryngeal nerve supplies the intrinsic muscles of the larynx; if the nerve is damaged by the tumour it will cause persistent hoarseness of the voice and may be the first symptom of the more serious condition.

25. Sympathetic trunk

Questions
- Which spinal nerves carry sympathetic nerve fibres?
- Which structures in the skin are involved in temperature regulation?
- Between which levels of the spinal cord do the sympathetic neurones lie?

Sympathetic nervous system

The sympathetic nervous system controls activities affecting the entire body, yet the cell bodies of sympathetic neurones are found *only* in the lateral grey of the thoracic spinal cord between **T1** and **L2**. How do their axons get to their destinations?

All that can be seen of the sympathetic system are the **sympathetic trunks** that lie on either side of the vertebral column from the base of the skull to the sacral region (Fig. 3.3.3, p. 31). The trunks connect a chain of segmental sympathetic ganglia where preganglionic fibres synapse with postganglionic neurones. The axons of postganglionic neurones are then distributed to the entire body surface in *every* spinal nerve (e.g. along intercostal nerves to supply the thoracic skin). In the head, where there are no *spinal* nerves, they are distributed along the arteries such as the internal carotid artery and its branches (Table 3.25.1).

Sympathetic supply routes
The axons of sympathetic neurones emerge from the spinal cord in the ventral roots of all the thoracic (intercostal nerves) and the first two lumbar spinal nerves. Almost immediately, they leave the spinal nerve and pass in a slender branch, the white ramus communicans (WRC), to reach a sympathetic ganglion where they synapse with their postganglionic neurones. The postganglionic axons rejoin the spinal nerve *via* the grey ramus communicans (GRC) and 'hitch hike' along the intercostal nerve to its distribution in the thoracic body wall (Fig. 3.25.1A).

Neurones supplying the skin of the upper limbs, head or neck (Fig. 3.25.1B) travel from the spinal cord in a thoracic spinal nerve and pass into the ganglion via the WRC. However, they pass straight through the ganglion, travel *up* the sympathetic trunk and eventually synapse in a cervical sympathetic ganglion. The postganglionic fibres either join cervical spinal nerves via their GRC and travel to destinations such as the upper limb or, if their destination is the head, they form a plexus on the surface of arteries such as the internal carotid and are distributed with the arterial branches. Likewise to reach the skin of the foot (Fig. 3.25.1C), preganglionic axons travel down the trunk, synapse in a ganglion at a lower level and join a lumbar spinal nerve. In this way, all the spinal nerves receive postganglionic sympathetic fibres for distribution to the structures in the skin and peripheral blood vessels.

Sympathetic neurones that supply thoracic viscera pass to sympathetic ganglia but do not synapse there (Fig. 3.25.1D). Instead, they pass directly in pulmonary or cardiac branches and synapse in the pulmonary and cardiac plexuses. Abdominal viscera are supplied in a similar way by preganglionic branches known as the **splanchnic nerves** (Fig. 3.25.1E). They pierce the crura of the diaphragm and synapse in the coeliac plexus, close to the abdominal viscera they supply.

Table 3.25.1 DISTRIBUTION OF SYMPATHETIC NERVES

Spinal levels	Preganglionic course	Synapse in	Viscera supplied	Some examples of stimulation
T1–T5	Pass up the sympathetic trunk	Cervical ganglia to internal carotid artery	Ciliary body of eye and skin of head and neck	Dilation of pupil; motor to levator palpebrae superiores; stimulates sweating, vasoconstriction of cutaneous vessels
T1–T5	Unnamed branches	Cardiac plexus	Heart	Increases cardiac output; dilatation of coronary arteries
T2–T4	Unnamed branches	Pulmonary plexus	Lungs	Dilatation of bronchioles
T2–T5	Pass up the sympathetic trunk	Cervical ganglia to brachial plexus	Upper limb skin	Stimulates sweating; vasoconstriction of cutaneous vessels
T6–T12	Greater, lesser and least splanchnic nerves	Coeliac ganglion	Abdominal viscera	Inhibition of secretion and peristalsis
L1–L2	Lumbar splanchnic nerves	Mesenteric ganglia	Pelvic viscera	Ejaculation
T11–L2	Pass down the sympathetic trunk	Lumbar ganglia to lumbar and sacral plexuses	Lower limb skin	Stimulates sweating; vasoconstriction of cutaneous vessels

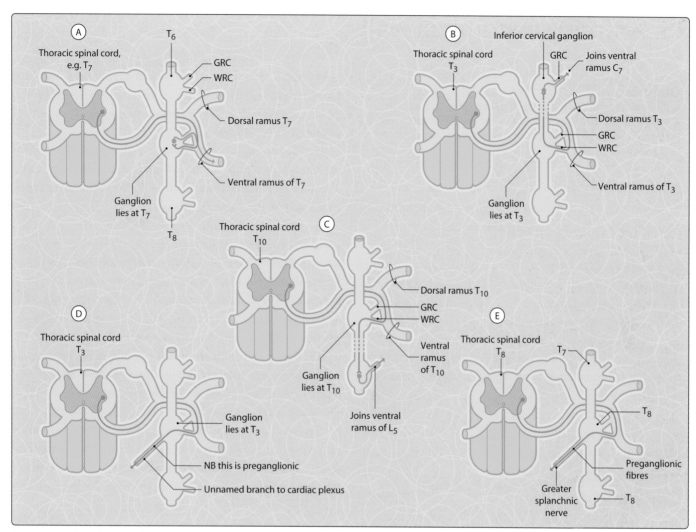

Fig. 3.25.1 Distribution of sympathetic postganglionic neurones: (A) in a spinal nerve to the thoracic body wall at the same level (e.g. sympathetic neurones from T$_7$ spinal segment supply a strip of skin at the level of the xiphoid); (B) in a spinal nerve to the body wall at a superior level (e.g. sympathetic neurones arising in spinal segment T$_3$ being distributed to the upper limb in C7); (C) in a spinal nerve to the body wall at an inferior level (e.g. sympathetic neurones arising in spinal segment T$_{10}$ being distributed to the lower limb in L5); (D) in unnamed branches to the cardiac plexus; (E) via the greater splanchnic nerve to the viscera of the abdomen (e.g. via the coeliac plexus). GRC, grey ramus communicans; WRC, white ramus communicans.

26. Anterior abdominal wall

Questions
- Which abdominal organs can be damaged in rib fractures?
- Which dermatome lies at the level of the umbilicus?
- What is the nerve supply of the anterior abdominal wall?

The abdominal or peritoneal cavity is separated from the thorax by the diaphragm. It is continuous with the pelvic cavity and is separated from the perineum by the pelvic diaphragm (Fig. 3.1.3, p. 27). The body wall is entirely muscular anteriorly and laterally; posteriorly it is supported by the lumbar spine and bony pelvis. The rib cage overlaps some upper abdominal organs (e.g. liver, spleen, kidneys) and others lie within the bony pelvis (e.g. bladder, uterus).

Figure 3.26.1 shows the nine regions. Four quadrants are often used in clinical examinations and a good knowledge of surface markings is essential.

The fatty superficial fascia varies in thickness (Camper's fascia). The deep fascia is known clinically as Scarper's fascia. Transversalis fascia lies between transversus abdominis and parietal peritoneum.

Muscles
The four muscles of the anterior abdominal wall fill the region between the costal margin and the superior parts of the bony pelvis (Fig. 3.26.2). They are important in flexing, twisting and lateral flexion of the trunk. Their contraction increases pressure in the abdominal cavity during activities such as lifting, coughing and defecation.

Rectus abdominis is a strap-like muscle on either side of the midline attached to the costal margin and the pubic symphysis. The muscle is subdivided by three or four tendinous intersections to form the enviable six pack!

The other three muscles are sheet-like muscles and attach superiorly to the costal margins and posterolaterally to lumbar fascia. Anteriorly, the muscles form the **rectus sheath** (Fig. 3.26.3). **External oblique** is the most superficial muscle; its fibres run downwards and medially from the lower eight ribs. The aponeurosis forms the anterior wall of the rectus sheath. Its inferior margin is suspended between its attachments to the pubic tubercle and the anterior superior iliac spine, forming the inguinal ligament. **Internal oblique** fibres run down and laterally, its aponeurosis splits to form the anterior and posterior walls of the rectus sheath. Inferiorly, its tendinous fibres arch from the inguinal ligament to the pubic tubercle and with similar fibres from the transversus abdominis form the **conjoint tendon** (p. 78). **Transversus abdominis** is the deepest muscle; its fibres run horizontally. Inferiorly it contributes to the conjoint tendon.

Rectus sheath
The rectus sheath is formed by the tendinous aponeuroses of the abdominal muscles. Medially, the sheaths meet at the **linea alba** and the lateral edge forms the **linea semilunaris,** which intersects the 9th costal cartilage (transpyloric plane). Above the umbilicus, the sheath has an anterior and a posterior wall, but inferiorly the posterior wall is absent leaving rectus abdominis in direct contact with the transversalis fascia (Fig. 3.26.3). The **arcuate line** is the inferior margin of the posterior wall.

Nerve supply
Intercostal nerves T_7–T_{12} pass forwards between the internal oblique and transversus abdominis muscles to supply the muscles and skin of the anterior abdominal wall. They pierce the rectus sheath, supply the rectus muscle and terminate as anterior cutaneous branches to the skin of the abdomen: T_7 supplying skin at the level of the xiphoid; T_{10} that at the level of the umbilicus; T_{12} the suprapubic area; and L_1 dividing to give the **iliohypogastric nerve** (to skin over the pubis) and the **ilioinguinal nerve** (to the anterior part of the scrotum and root of the penis/labia and clitoris).

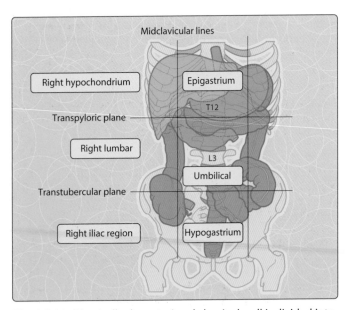

Midclavicular lines

Right hypochondrium

Epigastrium

T12

Transpyloric plane

Right lumbar

L3

Umbilical

Transtubercular plane

Right iliac region

Hypogastrium

Fig. 3.26.1 Classically the anterior abdominal wall is divided into nine regions by the transpyloric and transtubercular planes and the two vertical lines shown in this figure. The positions of the viscera are approximate.

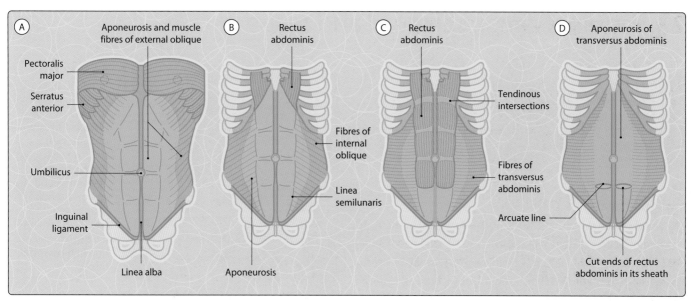

Fig. 3.26.2 Muscles of the abdominal wall from superficial to deep. (A) External oblique; (B) internal oblique; (C) rectus abdominis; (D) posterior wall of the rectus sheath.

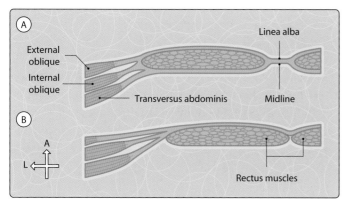

Fig. 3.26.3 Horizontal sections to show how the abdominal muscles contribute to the rectus sheath: (A) between the costal margin and the umbilicus; (B) below the arcuate line.

Blood supply

Intercostal arteries supply the wall laterally (Fig. 3.26.4). Anteriorly, the rectus sheath contains the superior epigastric artery (terminal branch of the internal thoracic artery; p. 56), which anastomoses with the inferior epigastric artery (branch of the external iliac; p. 110). The superior epigastric veins drain via the internal thoracic and subclavian veins to the superior vena cava and the inferior epigastric via the external iliac to the inferior vena cava. (See p. 85 for portosystemic anastomoses.)

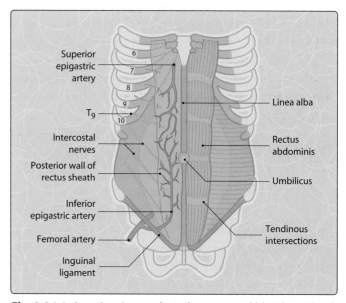

Fig. 3.26.4 Anterior view to show the nerve and blood supply of the anterior abdominal wall. Rectus abdominis is removed on the left to show the posterior wall of the rectus sheath.

 ABDOMINAL INCISIONS

Major incisions include:
- **median**: the linea alba is relatively bloodless and nerveless
- **paramedian**: an incision is made in the rectus sheath and the rectus is displaced *laterally* to avoid damage to the nerves entering the sheath laterally
- **through the sheet muscles**: damage to nerves can cause muscle paralysis and atrophy, with increased risk of hernia.

27. Inguinal canal, scrotum and testis

Questions
- What are the coverings of the spermatic cord?
- What is the lymphatic drainage of the testis?
- Where does an inguinal hernia lie in relation to the pubic tubercle?

Inguinal canal

The **inguinal canal** lies in the lower abdominal wall. In males, it transmits the **spermatic cord** and is a site of weakness where inguinal hernias may occur. In females, the canal is much smaller and does not usually cause problems (but see femoral hernia, p. 115).

What seems to be a 'design fault' is, in fact, a unique requirement of spermatogenesis, which requires a testicular temperature 2°C lower than normal body temperature. The testis begins its development high in the abdomen but descends during fetal life and around the time of birth pushes through the anterior abdominal wall dragging behind it its **vas deferens** and *original* blood supply, nerves and lymphatics in the **spermatic cord**. Postnatally, the testes lie in the scrotum connected to the abdomen via the spermatic cord and maintained at a temperature of 35°C, perfect for sperm production.

In females, the ovaries *begin* to migrate inferiorly but become fixed in the pelvic cavity (p. 104). The female equivalent to the spermatic cord is the **round ligament of the uterus**, which passes through the inguinal canal and attaches to the labia majora (homologous to the scrotum).

Understanding the anatomy of the inguinal canal is the key to understanding **inguinal herniae**. Figure 3.27.1 shows the structures as you would dissect them from superficial to deep. Then think of the route that the testis would have taken to understand the arrangement of the layers of the spermatic cord, i.e. from deep to superficial.

The canal is approximately 4 cm long and begins at the **deep inguinal ring** 2 cm above the femoral pulse at the inguinal ligament as a gap in the transversalis fascia. It passes medially under the tendinous arch formed by transversus abdominis and internal oblique and ends above and medial to the pubic tubercle at the **superficial inguinal ring**, which is a deficit in external oblique.

- Its floor is the inguinal ligament, which is the inferior border of external oblique (J shaped in cross-section).
- The anterior wall is the external oblique, reinforced laterally over the deep ring by the internal oblique.
- The posterior wall is transversalis fascia, reinforced medially by the conjoint tendon (internal oblique and transversus fibres).

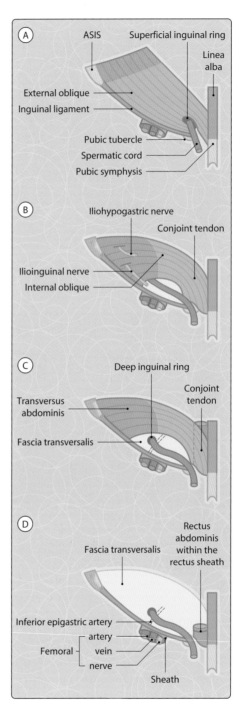

Fig. 3.27.1 The inguinal canal. (A) Superficial inguinal ring in external oblique; (B) internal oblique with branches of L_1; (C) transversus abdominis and conjoint tendon lying anterior to rectus abdominis; (D) deep inguinal ring in transversalis fascia.

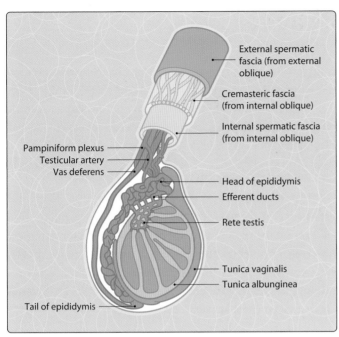

External spermatic fascia (from external oblique)

Cremasteric fascia (from internal oblique)

Internal spermatic fascia (from internal oblique)

Pampiniform plexus
Testicular artery
Vas deferens

Head of epididymis
Efferent ducts

Rete testis

Tunica vaginalis
Tunica albunginea

Tail of epididymis

Fig. 3.27.2 Coverings and content of the spermatic cord. The testis is sectioned to show its internal structure.

- Its roof is the conjoint tendon, which is the fusion of internal oblique and transversus abdominis.

Spermatic cord

Coverings

As the testis migrates, it carries with it the layers of the anterior abdominal wall through which it passes and these form the **coverings of the spermatic cord** (Fig. 3.27.2). Thus the *innermost* covering is derived from the *first* abdominal layer through which the testis must pass (NB transversus abdominis does not give rise to a covering because the testis passes beneath it).

1. Transversalis fascia gives rise to the **internal spermatic fascia**
2. Internal oblique extends to form **cremaster muscle** and **cremasteric fascia**
3. External oblique forms the **external spermatic fascia**.

Contents

The contents of the cord are:

- **vas deferens** continues into the abdomen posterior to the bladder and carries spermatozoa from the testis into the prostatic urethra (p. 102)
- **testicular artery** (branch of the aorta), artery to the ductus and artery to cremaster muscle
- **pampiniform venous plexus** around the testicular artery acts as a heat exchanger cooling the arterial blood supply to

the testis; the testicular veins drain to the inferior vena cava on the right and renal vein on the left

- **genital branch of the genitofemoral nerve** (L₁) passes through the deep inguinal ring, supplies the cremaster muscle and carries **sympathetic fibres** to dartos
- **lymphatics** drain to *aortic* nodes
- **processus vaginalis** is the obliterated remains of the peritoneal connection with the tunica vaginalis of the testis.

Scrotum and testis

The testes lie at the end of the spermatic cord in the scrotal sac, which consists of thin skin, the **dartos muscle** (which contracts in response to cold, wrinkling the skin of the scrotum) and a layer of fascia (Colles' fascia) that is continuous with Scarpa's fascia of the anterior abdominal wall. Remember that the scrotum is part of the body wall and receives a blood supply from the adjacent femoral vessels and a nerve supply from the ilioinguinal (L₁) and perineal nerves.

The testis is surrounded anteriorly and laterally by a serous sac, the **tunica vaginalis**, which is the remains of a pouch of the peritoneum that descends with the testis into the scrotum. The descent of the testis is 'guided' by a fibrous band of tissue, the **gubernaculum testis**, which attaches the inferior pole of the testis to the scrotal sac.

The testes consist of very extensive, coiled **seminiferous tubules**, which produce spermatozoa. The tubules are divided into lobes by connective tissue derived from the tough outer coat (**tunica albuginea**). Posteriorly, the tubules join to form the **rete testis** and **efferent tubules**; these empty into the head of the epididymis (Fig. 3.27.2). Sperm are stored in the head, body and tail of the epididymis. At ejaculation, sperm are propelled along the muscular vas deferens to empty into the prostatic urethra.

 TYPES OF INGUINAL HERNIA

Indirect inguinal hernia bulges through the deep inguinal ring into the canal. It may be large enough to emerge through the superficial ring just above the pubic tubercle and appearing as a scrotal swelling. It lies lateral to the inferior epigastric artery.

Direct inguinal hernia is caused by weakness of the conjoint tendon and is commoner in mature men. The hernia bulges through the conjoint tendon between the deep ring and the midline and lies medial to the inferior epigastric artery.

Congenital inguinal hernia results from developmental failure of the processus vaginalis to separate from the peritoneal cavity. The scrotum may contain coils of intestine.

28. Peritoneum and peritoneal cavity

Questions
- Which part of the embryonic gut has both a dorsal and a ventral mesentery?
- Where does the lesser sac lie in relation to the stomach?
- What structure develops in the inferior free margin of the ventral mesentery?

During embryonic development, the lungs become enclosed by the pleural membranes and the parietal peritoneum simply lines the abdominal cavity and the gut tube invaginates into it. Strictly speaking, the peritoneal cavity contains only a lubricating film of fluid between the parietal and visceral layers. The arrangement of the visceral layer becomes complex as it surrounds the intricately folded gut tube, liver and spleen. The blood supply, nerves and lymphatics of the viscera have to pass from the posterior abdominal wall within a **mesentery** (in the embryo this is called the *dorsal* mesentery). Viscera with a mesentery are mobile; the degree of mobility depends on the length of the mesentery (Table 3.28.1).

By the third week of gestation, the gut can be divided into three regions, the **foregut, midgut** (still opening ventrally into the yolk sac at this stage) and **hindgut**. Between the thorax and the abdomen, the foregut is closely related to the developing **septum transversum**, which gives rise to the diaphragm, liver and **ventral mesentery**; the last connects the foregut to the ventral body wall. The midgut and hindgut do not develop a ventral mesentery and so have a lower free edge in which the gall bladder and bile duct will develop (Fig. 3.28.1).

Lesser and greater sacs
During weeks 4 and 5 of embryonic development, differential growth of the foregut swings the stomach to the left and the liver enlarges on the right. The space posterior to the stomach is the **lesser sac** or **omental bursa**, which is connected to the **greater sac** (which is the rest of the peritoneal cavity) via a narrow opening, the epiploic foramen. Surgical incisions of the anterior abdominal enter the greater sac.

Lesser omentum and greater omentum
The **lesser omentum** (mesentery) develops from the embryonic ventral mesentery and connects the lesser curvature of the stomach and proximal duodenum with the liver. It has an inferior free border in which the bile duct develops and,

Table 3.28.1 MESENTERIES AND ASSOCIATED ARTERIES

Viscus	Mesenteries	Arteries
Stomach	Lesser omentum	Left and right gastric arteries and, in its free border, the hepatic artery, portal vein and bile duct
	Anterior layer of greater omentum	Left and right gastroepiploic arteries
Transverse colon	Transverse mesocolon	Middle colic
	Posterior layer of greater omentum	Middle colic
Spleen	Lienorenal ligament	Splenic artery
	Gastrosplenic ligament	Short gastric and left gastroepiploic arteries
Liver	Falciform ligament	Obliterated umbilical vein
	Lesser omentum	As for stomach
Small intestine	Mesentery of the small intestine	Superior mesenteric
Sigmoid colon	Sigmoid mesocolon	Sigmoid artery

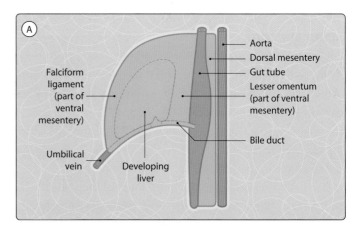

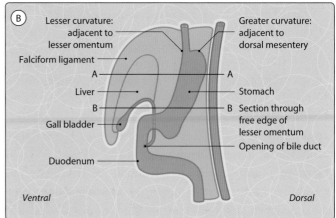

Fig. 3.28.1 Arrangement of the dorsal and ventral mesenteries of the foregut in sagittal section. (A) Early; (B) late.

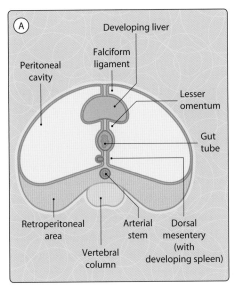

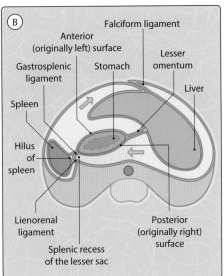

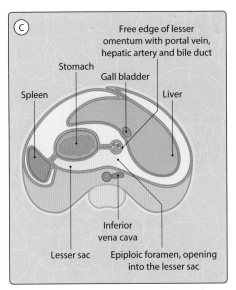

Fig. 3.28.2 Transverse section of the fetal abdomen showing the peritoneal arrangement of the foregut. (A) Early stage; (B) above the free edge of the ventral mesentery or lesser omentum (A/A in Fig. 3.28.1B); (C) through the free edge of the ventral mesentery (B/B in Fig. 3.28.1B).

together with the hepatic artery and portal vein, it forms the anterior border of the epiploic foramen (Fig. 3.28.2C).

The **greater omentum** is a large double layer that covers the intestines anteriorly like an apron (Fig. 3.28.3, see also Figs 3.31.1 and 3.31.2). It contains fat, which can be considerable. It develops as a downgrowth of peritoneum from the greater curvature of the stomach and the first part of the duodenum before folding back upwards to enclose the transverse colon. The lesser sac invaginates from behind into the fold and the layers fuse together.

Anterior abdominal wall

There are three peritoneal folds on the deep surface:

- one **median umbilical ligament** from the apex of the bladder to the umbilicus
- two **medial umbilical ligaments** representing obliterated umbilical arteries
- one **ligamentum teres**, the remnant of the obliterated umbilical vein; it lies in the **falciform ligament**, which forms the free inferior margin of the ventral mesentery between the liver and the anterior abdominal wall.

The peritoneal cavity

The mesentery of the transverse colon divides the peritoneal cavity into the **supracolic compartment**, containing the stomach, liver and spleen, and the **infracolic compartment**, containing the small intestine, colon and rectum. **Paracolic gutters** connect the supra- and infracolic compartments on either side.

The abdominal cavity (and, therefore, the peritoneal cavity) is kidney shaped in transverse section. On either side of the lumbar

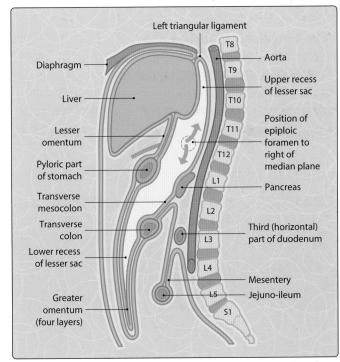

Fig. 3.28.3 Median sagittal section of the fetal abdomen to show the formation of the greater omentum.

spine are deep **paravertebral gutters** in which lie the ascending (right) and descending (left) limbs of the colon together with the kidneys and suprarenal glands. Lordosis of the lumbar spine means that free fluid gravitates into the *upper* abdomen.

The enormous surface area of the peritoneum has several implications: infection or malignant disease can spread rapidly; folds create sacs into which pus or fluid can collect; and treatment such as peritoneal dialysis is effective.

29. Arteries of the abdomen

Questions

- What is the blood supply of the lower one-third of the oesophagus?
- In general, what is the embryonic origin of the structures supplied by the superior mesenteric artery?
- Which structures does the inferior mesenteric artery supply?

The abdominal aorta is the continuation of the thoracic aorta (Fig. 3.29.1). It passes with the thoracic duct and azygos vein slightly to the left of the midline behind the median arcuate ligament of the diaphragm at the level of T12. It lies retroperitoneally on the lumbar vertebral bodies and divides at the level of L4 into the **common iliac arteries**, which supply the pelvis and lower limbs.

When you are learning about the aortic branches, think of them from posterior to anterior (Fig. 3.29.1).

Paired posterior branches

Pairs of intercostal arteries arise from the thoracic aorta and supply the thoracic wall. The subcostal artery lies below the 12th rib and it supplies the abdominal wall. Inferiorly, paired lumbar arteries supply the posterior abdominal body wall and the lumbar region of the spinal cord.

Paired visceral branches

The visceral branches are quite variable; the renal arteries arise at L1/L2, the adrenal arteries at L1 and the gonadal arteries at L2.

Unpaired anterior visceral branches

The coeliac trunk

The **coeliac trunk** (axis) supplies the embryonic foregut and structures that develop in its mesenteries (stomach, liver, spleen, most of the pancreas, greater and lesser omenta). It arises from the anterior aspect of the aorta 0.5 cm below the diaphragm at the level of T12 and quickly divides to give three important terminal branches (Fig. 3.29.2):

- left gastric artery
- splenic artery
- common hepatic artery.

The **left gastric artery** runs superiorly in the posterior wall of the lesser sac. It divides to give **oesophageal branches**, which pass through the oesophageal opening in the diaphragm to supply the lower one-third of the oesophagus. The left gastric artery supplies the lesser curvature of the stomach before anastomosing with the right gastric artery.

The **splenic artery** has a characteristically tortuous course in the posterior wall of the lesser sac. It passes to the left along the superior border of the pancreas as far as the upper pole of

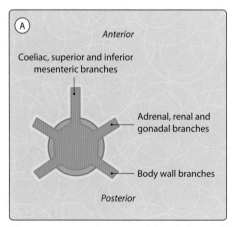

Fig. 3.29.1 Anterior view of the abdominal aorta and its branches. (A) Diagram to show layout of branches; (B) anterior view.

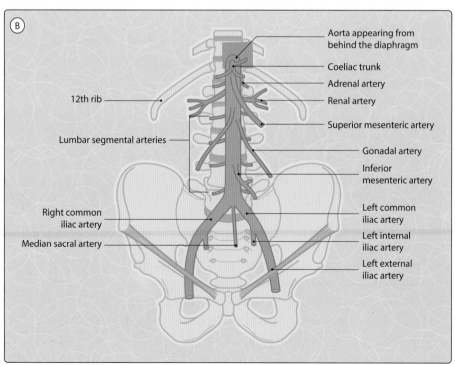

the kidney before entering the lienorenal ligament to reach the spleen. It also gives short **gastric arteries** to the fundus of the stomach and the **left gastroepiploic artery**, which supplies the greater curvature of the stomach.

The **common hepatic artery** passes inferiorly and to the right in the posterior wall of the lesser sac towards the first part of the duodenum, where it divides into branches to the duodenum (**gastroduodenal**) and stomach (**right gastric**). The main trunk, the **hepatic artery proper**, curves anteriorly to lie in the free border of the lesser omentum (anterior margin of the epiploic foramen) with the hepatic portal vein and bile duct (Fig. 3.28.2C, p. 81). Just before entering the porta hepatis, the artery divides into right and left hepatic arteries. The **gastroduodenal artery** passes behind the first part of the duodenum and divides into the superior pancreaticoduodenal and right gastroepiploic arteries.

The mesenteric arteries

The **superior mesenteric artery** supplies the embryonic midgut (distal duodenum, uncinate process of the pancreas, small intestine and colon as far as the splenic flexure). It arises at L1 and passes over the left renal vein behind the neck of the pancreas, over the uncinate process and anterior to the third part of the duodenum (Fig. 3.29.3). It passes to the right and from the mesentery of the small intestine gives the following branches:

- inferior pancreaticoduodenal artery, which anastomoses with the superior pancreaticoduodenal artery
- ileocaecal artery, which passes anterior to the right ureter and gonadal vessels to supply the caecum
- jejunal and ileal branches (12–15 in total), which supply the small bowel
- right colic artery, which supplies the ascending colon
- middle colic artery, which supplies the proximal two-thirds of the transverse colon.

The **inferior mesenteric artery** supplies the hindgut (descending colon, sigmoid, colon, rectum and upper part of the anal canal). It arises at L3, passes downwards and to the left crossing the left common iliac. It divides within the mesocolon to give:

- **left colic artery**, which supplies the remainder of the colon
- **sigmoid branches**, which supply the most distal portion of the descending colon and sigmoid colon
- **superior rectal artery**, which passes behind the rectum to anastomose with middle and inferior rectal arteries.

 AORTIC ANEURYSM

Aortic aneurysm is caused by local weakness of the wall of the aorta that leads to an enlargement at that point; this may eventually rupture if not repaired. It can be repaired by opening the aneurysm and inserting a Dacron graft.

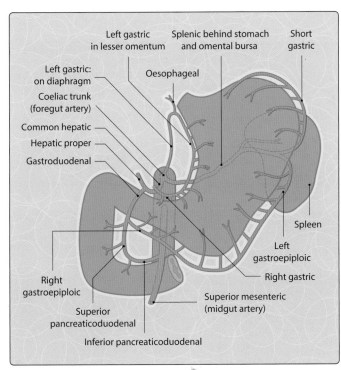

Fig. 3.29.2 Branches of the coeliac trunk (foregut artery).

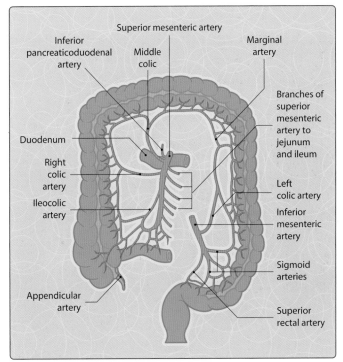

Fig. 3.29.3 Branches of the superior and inferior mesenteric arteries (mid- and hindgut arteries).

30. Veins and lymphatics of the abdomen

Questions
- What is the venous drainage of the intestines?
- Where does the inferior vena cava lie in relation to the epiploic foramen?
- What is the significance of portosystemic anastomoses?

Inferior vena cava

The inferior vena cava (IVC) returns venous blood from the abdomen and lower limbs to the *right* atrium (Fig. 3.30.1). In the abdomen, therefore, it lies to the *right* of the aorta. It is formed from the common iliac veins and its main tributaries are renal, adrenal, gonadal and hepatic veins. Importantly, *it does not drain the intestine*. The IVC lies in the posterior wall of the epiploic foramen and is embedded in the bare area of the liver anterior to the right adrenal gland. It pierces the central tendon of the diaphragm at the level of T8 (along with the right phrenic nerve).

Portal system

The **hepatic portal vein** carries venous blood from the intestines, spleen and pancreas to the liver, where nutrients absorbed by the gut can be metabolized. The portal vein forms behind the neck of the pancreas from the union of the splenic vein with the superior mesenteric veins (Fig. 3.30.2). The portal vein passes behind the first part of the duodenum lying in front

of the IVC and enters the anterior free margin of the lesser omentum (epiploic foramen). At the **porta hepatis,** it divides into right and left branches in the same fashion as the hepatic artery and bile duct.

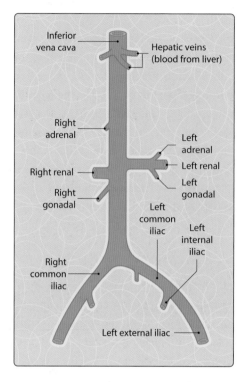

Fig. 3.30.1 Anterior view of the inferior vena cava and its major tributaries.

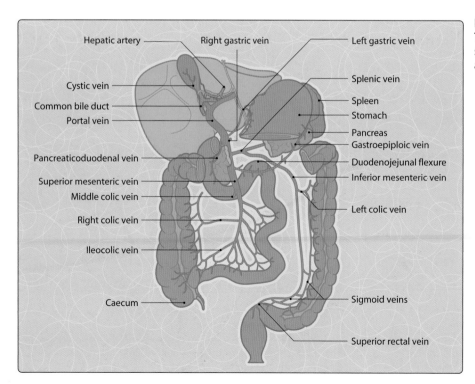

Fig. 3.30.2 Portal vein and its tributaries. The liver is lifted to show the visceral surface. The body of the stomach, pancreas and transverse colon have been removed.

Lymphatic drainage

The anterior abdominal wall is divided into two regions:

- above the umbilicus, which drains to the axillary nodes
- below the umbilicus, which drains to the superficial inguinal nodes.

Preaortic nodes lie around the three anterior visceral branches of the aorta and drain the territory of these arteries, i.e. most of the intestines, liver, gall bladder, spleen and pancreas (e.g. the stomach drains to coeliac nodes). Lymph drains from the pre-aortic nodes via intestinal trunks to the cisterna chyli (Fig. 3.30.3).

Para-aortic nodes are arranged around the lateral branches of the aorta and drain corresponding territories, i.e. kidneys, adrenals and gonads. The common iliac nodes draining the pelvis and lower limbs also drain to these nodes. Lumbar trunks carry lymph to the cisterna chyli.

Cisterna chyli

The cisterna chyli is a thin-walled lymphatic sac about 5 cm long that lies anterior to the vertebral bodies of L1 and L2 at the inferior end of the thoracic duct. It receives lymph from the intestinal and lumbar trunks before entering the thoracic duct (p. 69).

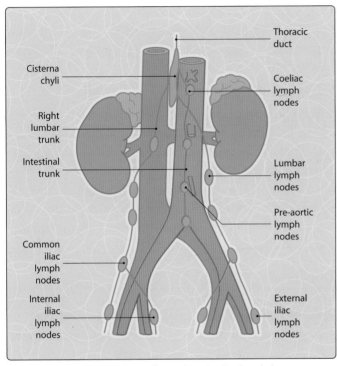

Fig. 3.30.3 Major lymph trunks and nodes in the abdomen.

 PORTOSYSTEMIC ANASTOMOSES

All venous blood from the intestine drains via the portal vein to the liver. Liver disease (e.g. cirrhosis) may obstruct the direct pathway through the liver and cause venous congestion (**portal hypertension**). The rise in pressure in the portal vein causes blood to be shunted into venous connections between the systemic and portal systems. The major sites of porto-systemic anastomosis are:

- lower one-third of the oesophagus: left gastric veins (portal) connect with tributaries of the azygos system (systemic)
- anterior abdominal wall: paraumbilical veins (portal) connect with epigastric veins (systemic) causing enlarged veins that radiate from the umbilicus; these are called caput medusae.
- anal canal: superior rectal (portal) with middle and inferior rectal (systemic).
- bare area of the liver: the connections between the portal system and the phrenic veins are clinically insignificant.

31. Oesophagus, stomach and duodenum

Questions
- Which structures form the stomach bed?
- At what vertebral level does the pylorus lie?
- Why are the relations of the duodenum important?

Oesophagus

The embryonic foregut comprises the pharynx, oesophagus, stomach and as far as the opening of the common bile duct into the second part of the duodenum.

The **abdominal oesophagus** is only 1 cm long; it enters the stomach at an acute angle to the fundus. It pierces the diaphragm just to the left of the median plane at the level of T10, supported by a muscular sling from the *right* crus of the diaphragm. The anterior and posterior vagal trunks accompany the oesophagus, together with branches of the left gastric vessels.

Stomach

The stomach lies between the oesophagus and the duodenum across the supracolic compartment from upper left to lower right (Fig. 3.31.1). It is a J- or C-shaped muscular sac with anterior and posterior surfaces and borders known as the **greater** and **lesser curvatures**. Its internal surface is thrown into folds (rugae).

Undefined muscle fibres in the region of the cardia help to prevent reflux of the acid contents of the stomach into the oesophagus. The **pyloric sphincter** is a palpable thickening of circular muscle that controls the passage of gastric contents into the duodenum. It lies at the level of L1 (the transpyloric plane) to the right of the midline.

The lesser omentum is attached to the lesser curvature of the stomach and the greater omentum to the greater curvature (see Fig. 3.31.2).

The stomach has a very rich arterial supply from all three branches of the coeliac trunk (p. 82). They form anastomoses on the greater and lesser curvatures. Gastric veins drain to the portal vein. The lower third of the oesophagus is an important site of portosystemic anastomosis between the left gastric and azygos veins (p. 85).

Relations

Anteriorly the stomach is overlapped by the left lobe of the liver and on the right by the diaphragm and costal margins. A small central area is in contact with the peritoneum posterior to the rectus sheath (Fig. 3.31.3).

Posteriorly the lesser sac separates the stomach from the **stomach bed,** which consists of the pancreas, mesentery of the transverse colon, spleen, splenic artery, left kidney, suprarenal gland and diaphragm (Fig. 3.31.4).

Duodenum

The small intestine consists of the duodenum, jejunum and ileum. The first part of the small intestine, the duodenum, is a C-shaped tube about 25 cm long (Figs 3.29.2 and 3.32.4). Only the

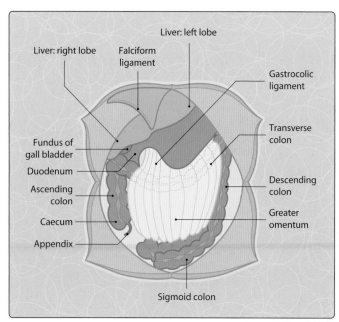

Fig. 3.31.1 Abdominal wall opened to show the position of the stomach and the greater omentum.

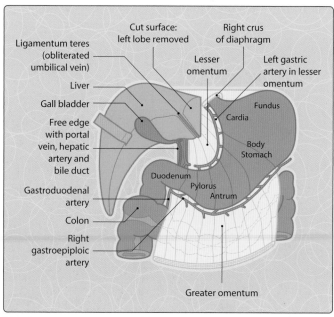

Fig. 3.31.2 Anterior view of the stomach with the left lobe of the liver removed.

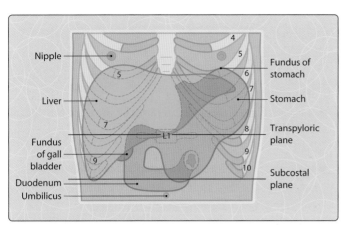

Fundus
of gall
bladder

Nipple

Liver

Duodenum
Umbilicus

4

5

5

6

7

7

L1

9

9

8

9

10

Fundus of
stomach

Stomach

Transpyloric
plane

Subcostal
plane

Fig. 3.31.3 Surface projections and markings of the liver, stomach and duodenum.

first part is free to move with the stomach, the remainder is retroperitoneal. It is described in four parts.

■ The **first (superior) part** (5 cm) passes posteriorly from the pylorus to the right of the vertebral column. It is overlapped by the liver and gall bladder and lies on the bile duct and right kidney. It is susceptible to peptic ulceration, which can affect adjacent structures.

■ The **second (descending) part** (7.5 cm) passes posteriorly and inferiorly curving round the head of the pancreas. The common opening of the bile and main pancreatic ducts, the **major duodenal papilla**, lies on the posteromedial wall (Fig. 3.32.4, p. 89). If it is present, the opening of an accessory pancreatic duct lies superiorly (**minor duodenal papilla**). The transverse colon lies anteriorly (Fig. 3.32.3).

■ The **third (inferior) part** (10 cm) passes to the left, anterior to the inferior vena cava and aorta at L3 and is itself posterior to the root of 'the mesentery' (Fig. 3.32.2).

■ The **fourth (ascending) part** (2.5 cm) passes superiorly and anteriorly, is continuous with the jejunum at the duodeno-jejunal flexure at L2 and is usually related to the inferior mesenteric vein (Fig. 3.30.2).

Blood, lymphatic and nerve supply

Blood supply is from the superior pancreaticoduodenal artery (branch of the hepatic artery) and the inferior pancreaticoduodenal artery (branch of the superior mesenteric arteries; p. 82).

Lymphatics in this region drain to the preaortic nodes, which may be surgically inaccessible.

The nerve supply is described on p. 97.

Relations

Relations of the duodenum are complex and important. Disease in one system can affect others. See the posterior relations in Fig. 3.33.2.

GASTROSCOPY

The mucosa of the oesophagus, stomach and duodenum can be visually inspected and a biopsy taken using a fibreoptic endoscope. There is an important transitional zone at the gastroesophageal junction between the stratified epithelial lining of the oesophagus and the simple columnar epithelium of the gut tube that begins with the gastric mucosa. There is no anatomical sphincter at this junction and acidic gastric contents may reflux causing ulceration of the lower one-third of the oesophagus, with an associated risk of adenocarcinoma in the long term.

Similar instruments make it possible to examine the duodenal mucosa and even the opening and lower segment of the bile duct. Gallstones impacted in the bile duct can now be crushed and removed endoscopically.

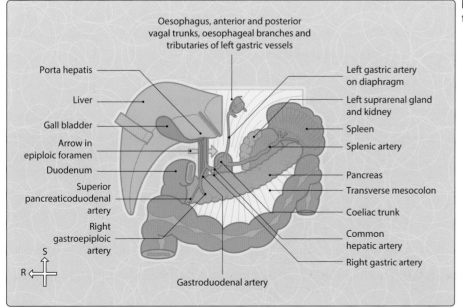

Porta hepatis

Liver

Gall bladder

Arrow in
epiploic foramen

Duodenum

Superior
pancreaticoduodenal
artery

Right
gastroepiploic
artery

Oesophagus, anterior and posterior
vagal trunks, oesophageal branches and
tributaries of left gastric vessels

Gastroduodenal artery

Left gastric artery
on diaphragm

Left suprarenal gland
and kidney

Spleen

Splenic artery

Pancreas

Transverse mesocolon

Coeliac trunk

Common
hepatic artery

Right gastric artery

S
R

Fig. 3.31.4 The structures that make up the stomach bed.

32. Liver and gall bladder

Questions
- What are the structures that enter the liver at the porta hepatis?
- What forms the posterior boundary of the epiploic foramen?
- How does blood flow through the liver?

Liver

The liver is the largest internal organ and has multiple metabolic activities, including the storage of glycogen and secretion of bile. It lies largely in the right hypochondrium and epigastric regions and extends into the left hypochondrium. It is wedge shaped with two surfaces separated by the inferior border. The **diaphragmatic surface** lies under the dome of the right hemi-diaphragm and is overlapped by the costal margin (Fig. 3.31.3). It is separated from the diaphragm by the **subphrenic recess** of the peritoneal cavity (Fig. 3.32.1). The **visceral surface** is covered by peritoneum except for the fossa of the gall bladder (Fig. 3.32.2A). There are superficial impressions for the right side of the stomach (gastric area), the duodenum (duodenal area), the gall bladder, the hepatic flexure of the colon (colic area) and the right kidney and suprarenal gland.

The peritoneal recess between the visceral surface and the right kidney is the **hepatorenal pouch (of Morison)** (Fig. 3.32.1).

The liver has four lobes. The large right and smaller left lobe are separated by the **falciform ligament** on the anterior surface (Fig. 3.32.2B). The **caudate** and **quadrate** lobes are best seen from the inferior surface (Fig. 3.32.2A) and which are helpfully described in terms of an H-shaped arrangement:

- the left limb is a deep cleft occupied anteriorly by the falciform ligament with the **ligamentum teres** and

posteriorly by part of the lesser omentum with the **ligamentum venosum**
- the right limb is formed anteriorly by the fossa for the gall bladder and posteriorly by the fossa for the inferior vena cava
- the cross-piece is the **porta hepatis;** the quadrate lobe lies anteriorly and the caudate lobe lies posteriorly, close to the inferior vena cava.

The structures that enter the **porta hepatis** are known as the **portal triad**. It consists of the right and left branches of the:

- **hepatic artery:** branches of the coeliac trunk, supplying the liver with oxygenated blood
- **hepatic portal vein:** returning venous blood carrying the products of digestion from the gut
- **hepatic ducts:** drain bile from the liver into the common hepatic duct.

The superficial lobes of the liver have no functional significance. However the branching pattern of the structures that enter the porta hepatis defines surgically important lobes and segments in a similar way to the bronchopulmonary segments of the lungs.

Peritoneal covering

The liver is enclosed in peritoneum except where it is in direct contact with the diaphragm (Fig. 3.32.2B). The margins of the **bare area** where the visceral peritoneum is reflected onto the undersurface of the diaphragm are known as the **coronary ligaments**. The **right** and **left triangular ligaments** are where the coronary ligaments fuse on either side. The liver is attached to the anterior abdominal wall by the falciform ligament. Inferiorly, the lesser omentum encloses the portal triad and passes to the lesser curvature of the stomach and the first part of the duodenum, to form the **hepatogastric** and **hepatoduodenal ligaments** (Fig. 3.32.3).

Blood, lymphatic and nerve supply

Blood from the hepatic portal vein and hepatic arteries mixes in the sinusoids of the liver and comes into intimate contact with hepatocytes for the exchange of nutrients and metabolic products. Blood then flows into tributaries of the hepatic vein before draining into the inferior vena cava, which passes through the bare area of the liver and pierces the diaphragm at T8 before entering the right atrium (Fig. 3.32.2A).

Lymphatics drain to hepatic nodes around the porta hepatis and thence to the preaortic nodes.

The nerve supply is described on p. 97.

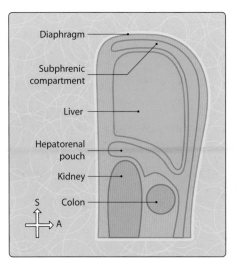

Fig. 3.32.1 Sagittal section of upper abdominal cavity to show the peritoneal recesses around the liver and kidney.

Diaphragm

Subphrenic compartment

Liver

Hepatorenal pouch

Kidney

Colon

S

A

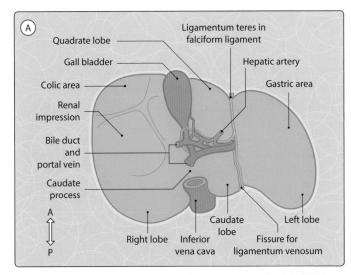

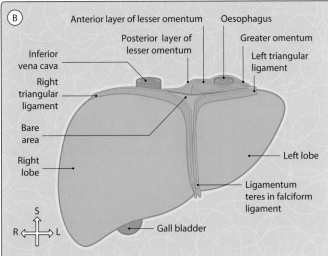

Fig. 3.32.2 The surface of the liver. (A) Visceral surface; (B) anterior surface.

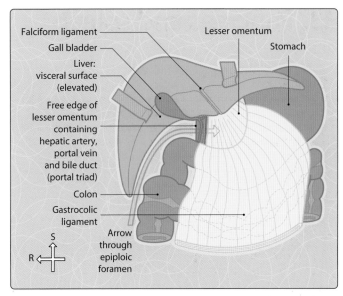

Fig. 3.32.3 The free border of the lesser omentum forming the anterior border of the epiploic foramen.

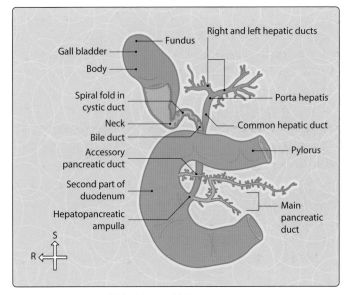

Fig. 3.32.4 The gall bladder and biliary tree.

Gall bladder

The gall bladder lies on the visceral surface of the liver behind the tip of the 9th costal cartilage. It stores about 50 ml of bile. Bile is released into the duodenum after a fatty meal (Fig. 3.32.4). Both the gall bladder and duct system are anatomically variable.

The biliary tree comprises the common hepatic duct (combining left and right hepatic ducts) and the cystic duct, which drain into the **common bile duct** (Fig. 3.32.4). The common bile duct runs in the free edge of the lesser omentum (Fig. 3.32.3), posterior to the duodenum and head of the pancreas before joining with the pancreatic duct at the hepatopancreatic ampulla (of Vater). The common opening empties into the second part of the duodenum (major duodenal papilla). The accessory pancreatic duct opens at the minor duodenal papilla (p. 90).

 OBSTRUCTIVE JAUNDICE

The narrowest part of the biliary tree, the hepatopancreatic ampulla, is a common site of blockage by a gallstone. If bile release is obstructed, excess bilirubin enters the blood, causing yellowing of the skin (jaundice) and dark urine; faeces become pale (through lack of the bile pigments) and fatty (because fat digestion is incomplete).

33. Pancreas and spleen

Questions
- What structures open into the hepatopancreatic ampulla? That is, why might gallstones cause pancreatitis?
- Which major structures lie on the posterior abdominal wall behind the pancreas?
- Why might a ruptured spleen present as left shoulder pain?

Pancreas

An understanding of early development helps to explain the relationships of the bile and pancreatic ducts (Fig. 3.33.1 and p. 89). The pancreas develops as ventral and dorsal outgrowths of the duodenum. The ventral pancreatic bud and the adjacent developing liver are carried around the duodenum, bringing their common duct close to the dorsal pancreatic bud. The pancreatic buds fuse; the ventral duct joins with the distal portion of the dorsal duct to form the main pancreatic duct and the remainder of the dorsal duct forms an accessory pancreatic duct.

Structure

The pancreas has a head, neck, body, tail and uncinate process (*uncus*, hook). The head and uncinate process lie within the curve of the duodenum and the body and tail pass across the upper part of the posterior abdominal wall to the hilum of the spleen, roughly in the transpyloric plane (Fig. 3.31.4). The pancreas is retroperitoneal (Fig. 3.33.1C) and consists of:

- **endocrine cells** (**islets of Langerhans**): secrete the hormones insulin and glucagon directly into the bloodstream
- **exocrine cells**: secrete a number of digestive enzymes into the pancreatic ducts, which open into the duodenum (Fig. 3.32.4)

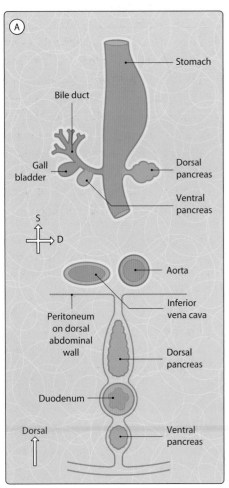
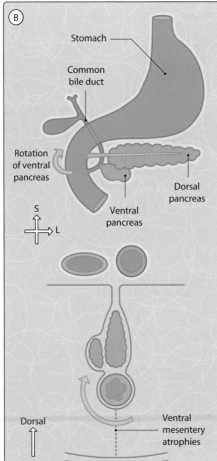
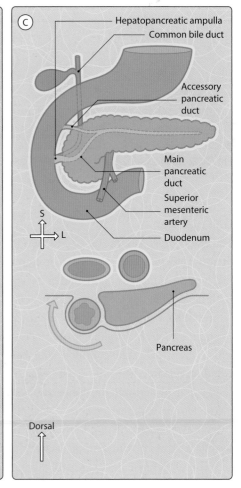

Fig. 3.33.1 Embryonic development of the pancreas and duodenum. Top row shows the formation and the bottom shows the transverse section. (A) Formation of the dorsal and ventral buds of the pancreas; (B) rotation of the ventral pancreas; (C) fusion of the buds to form the definitive pancreas and its ducts.

■ **main duct** begins at the tail and usually joins the **accessory duct** at the head before joining the bile duct as it pierces the posteromedial wall of the duodenum at the hepatopancreatic ampulla (major duodenal papilla); the accessory duct may open separately into the duodenum at the minor duodenal papilla (Fig. 3.33.1B,C).

Relations

The stomach and lesser sac lie anterior to the pancreas. Posteriorly are the inferior vena cava, the aorta, coeliac plexus, left kidney, suprarenal gland and their vessels (Fig. 3.33.2). The splenic vein crosses behind the gland, joining with the inferior mesenteric vein and then with the superior mesenteric vein to form the portal vein behind the neck (see Fig. 3.30.2). The splenic artery lies along the superior border. Note that the uncinate process 'hooks' behind the superior mesenteric artery. To the left, the tail lies in the lienorenal ligament and may touch the hilum of the spleen (Fig. 3.33.2).

Blood and nerve supply

Like the duodenum, the pancreas is supplied by the superior pancreaticoduodenal branch of the coeliac trunk and the inferior pancreaticoduodenal branch from the superior mesenteric arteries. The body of the pancreas is supplied by branches of the splenic artery. See p. 97 for nerve supply.

Spleen

The spleen develops in the embryonic dorsal mesentery from several masses of tissue, each with its own blood supply. It is connected to the posterior abdominal wall by the **splenorenal (lienorenal) ligament** and to the stomach by the **gastrosplenic ligament**. These ligaments form the left extremity of the lesser sac (Fig. 3.28.2B). Later, the inferior part of the gastrosplenic ligament enlarges to form the greater omentum.

Structure

The spleen is the largest mass of *lymphoid* tissue in the body (about the size of a clenched fist), but it does not receive afferent lymph vessels. It helps to mount an immunological response to blood-borne pathogens and is the major site of destruction of erythrocytes, white blood cells and platelets. Splenectomy leads to loss of defences against capsulated bacteria. The spleen has a fibrous capsule with a complete covering of peritoneum except at the hilum, where several branches of the splenic artery and associated veins enter its gastric surface (Fig. 3.33.2). The hilum normally lies in the transpyloric plane.

Relations

The spleen lies under the left dome of the diaphragm wedged between the stomach, left kidney and left colic flexure (hence splenic flexure). It is related to ribs 9, 10 and 11, with its long axis on the 10th rib, but is separated from them by the left costodiaphragmatic recess of the pleural cavity. Trauma to the lower left ribs may damage the highly vascular spleen and resulting haemorrhage can be life threatening. Free blood in the peritoneal cavity can irritate the peritoneal surface of the diaphragm, resulting in referred pain to the tip of the left shoulder (dermatome C_4). The normal spleen is not palpable. If it becomes enlarged, the notches on the superior margin may appear below the left costal margin at the 9th costal cartilage.

Blood supply

The splenic artery is a major branch of the coeliac trunk and has a characteristically tortuous course along the superior edge of the pancreas in the gastrosplenic ligament before entering the hilum of the spleen. The splenic vein drains to the portal vein.

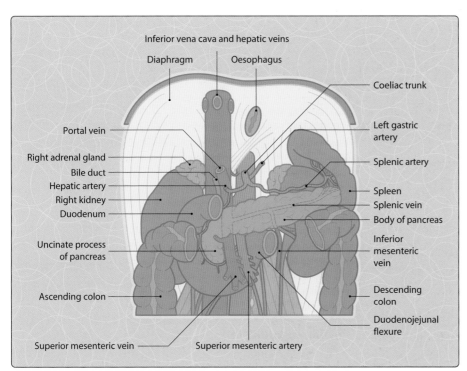

Inferior vena cava and hepatic veins
Diaphragm
Oesophagus
Coeliac trunk
Portal vein
Left gastric artery
Right adrenal gland
Splenic artery
Bile duct
Hepatic artery
Spleen
Right kidney
Splenic vein
Duodenum
Body of pancreas
Inferior mesenteric vein
Uncinate process of pancreas
Descending colon
Ascending colon
Duodenojejunal flexure
Superior mesenteric vein
Superior mesenteric artery

Fig. 3.33.2 Anterior view of the upper abdomen with the stomach, transverse colon, jejunum and ilium removed.

34. Mid- and hindgut

Questions
- How can you distinguish the ileum from the jejunum?
- Which branch of the aorta supplies the ascending colon?
- Which parts of the colon are suspended by a mesentery?

The **midgut** extends from the second part of the duodenum (duodenal papilla) to two-thirds of the way along the transverse colon and is supplied by the **superior mesenteric artery**. The **hindgut** includes the sigmoid colon to the upper half of the anal canal as far as the pectinate line and is supplied by the **inferior mesenteric artery**. Branches from each artery anastomose to form the marginal artery (Fig. 3.29.3). Both are drained by the hepatic portal vein. The midgut and hindgut lymphatic drainage is to nodes in their mesenteries before draining to the cysterna chyli via the preaortic nodes and intestinal trunks. (See p. 97 for the nerve supply.)

Development of the midgut

The midgut enlarges greatly during the fifth week of life and expands into the umbilical cord as a loop with the superior mesenteric artery as the axis between its cephalic and caudal limbs (Fig. 3.34.1A). At about the 10th week of gestation, the midgut rotates anticlockwise through 90 degrees and returns to the abdominal cavity. The cephalic limb leads and forms the proximal part of the small intestine, lying posterior to the superior mesenteric artery. The caudal limb returns to form the distal part of the ilium, caecum and colon as far as the distal two-thirds of the transverse colon. These movements push the hindgut to the left (Fig. 3.34.1B).

The boundary between the gut tube (embryonic endoderm) and the skin (embryonic ectoderm) lies at the white (pectinate) line in the anal canal. The anal canal is derived from endoderm and has a different blood supply, venous drainage and nerve supply to tissues derived from ectoderm (Table 3.38.1).

The small intestine

The small intestine lies in the infracolic compartment; it consists of the duodenum, jejunum and ileum (Fig. 3.34.2). The proximal part of the duodenum is retroperitoneal.

Mesentery

At the junction of the duodenum and jejunum (duodenojejunal flexure), the gut is suspended from the posterior abdominal wall by 'the mesentery'. Its line of origin passes obliquely from the duodenojejunal flexure to the right sacroiliac joint (Fig. 3.34.3).

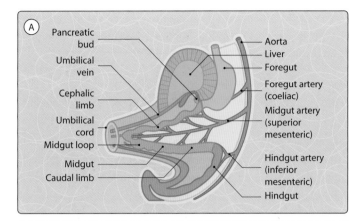

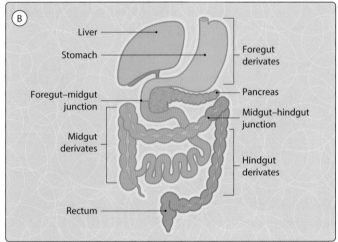

Fig. 3.34.1 Embryonic development of the gut. (A) Parts of the gut and their blood supply; (B) parts of the gut and their relative positions after rotation.

From this narrow (15 cm) origin, 'the mesentery' fans out dramatically, enclosing the superior mesenteric vessels, lymph nodes that drain the gut, and 6 m of small bowel. Internally, the small bowel has a huge surface area to facilitate absorption.

Jejunum and ileum

The jejunum (proximal two-fifths) and ileum (distal three-fifths) are both smooth walled but may be distinguished by the pattern of their blood supply from the superior mesenteric artery (Fig. 3.34.4). The coils of the jejunum tend to lie in the umbilical region and the ileum occupies the lower abdomen and pelvis. Large aggregations of subendothelial lymphoid tissue (**Peyer's patches**) occur in the ileum wall.

Caecum and colon

The caecum and colon (1.5 m in length) reabsorb water and propel faeces towards the anus. The external longitudinal muscle coat is concentrated into three bands (**teniae coli**); these

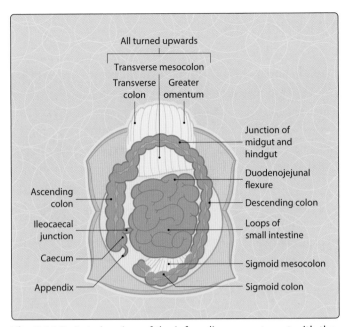

Fig. 3.34.2 Anterior view of the infracolic compartment with the greater omentum and the transverse mesocolon turned superiorly.

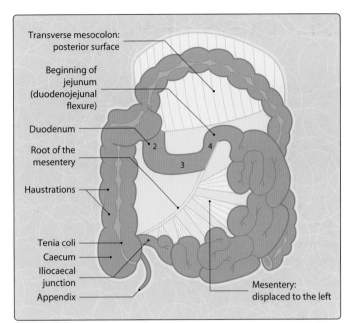

Fig. 3.34.3 Anterior view showing the origin of 'the mesentery'.

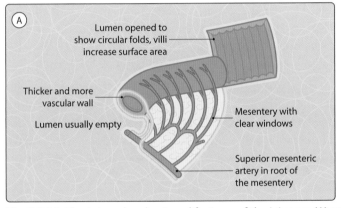

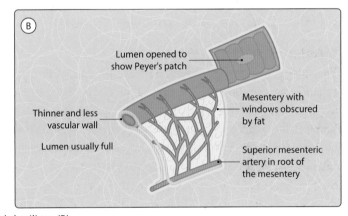

Fig. 3.34.4 The internal and external features of the jejunum (A) and the ilium (B).

are shorter than the gut tube, which, consequently, becomes gathered up into **sacculations** (**haustrations**) on the internal surface (Fig. 3.34.3). Characteristically, the colon has external fatty appendages: **appendices epiploicae**.

The **ascending colon** lies on the right and is retroperitoneal. At the right colic (hepatic) flexure, it turns transversely across the abdomen and is suspended by the **transverse mesocolon,** which allows the **transverse colon** to loop inferiorly. At the left colic (splenic) flexure, the **descending colon** turns inferiorly and becomes retroperitoneal. The **sigmoid colon** has a mesentery and meets the rectum in front of S3 (rectosigmoid junction).

The **appendix** is a narrow tube that usually lies behind the caecum (retrocaecal) and is 5–15 cm long. It has a small mesentery and the teniae coli converge to cover it. Its usual surface marking is McBurney's point, which lies two-thirds of

the way along the line from the umbilicus to the anterior superior iliac spine.

Rectum and anal canal

The rectum lies in the pelvis beginning opposite the third piece of the sacrum; it is 10–15 cm long and, at the tip of the coccyx, becomes the anal canal. The lower part of the rectum is expanded (ampulla) and bulges forwards. The teniae coli merge to form anterior and posterior longitudinal bands, throwing the internal lining into three horizontal folds. Peritoneum covers the front and sides of the upper one-third and the anterior of the middle one-third. The lower one-third is below the level of the peritoneum as it is reflected forwards onto the bladder in men and the uterus in women. The **anal canal** lies in the perineum.

35. Kidneys, ureters and adrenal glands

Questions
- Which part of the plural cavity lies posterior to the kidney?
- What are the bony landmarks that mark the course of the ureters?
- What type of tissue forms the medulla of the adrenal glands?

Development of the kidney

The kidneys develop in the pelvis and move *upwards* during development. The renal fascia is relatively open below along the line of their migration. As the kidneys ascend, inferior arteries degenerate as superior ones take over. Thus:

- the kidneys move up and down the posterior wall during breathing movements
- blood from a ruptured kidney accumulates first in the renal fascia and then tracks inferiorly towards the pelvis
- accessory renal arteries occur inferiorly (25% of individuals)
- failure to ascend results in persistent pelvic kidneys.

Kidneys

The kidneys lie retroperitoneally on either side of the vertebral column between T12 and L3; because of the position of the liver, the right kidney is about 1 cm lower than the left. Each is enclosed by a tough **capsule** and surrounded by perinephric **fat.** The **renal fascia** holds the kidney in position and separately encloses the adrenal glands above (Fig. 3.35.1).

It is important to note that the kidneys are overlapped by the 12th ribs and that they are directly related to the diaphragm, which separates them from the costodiaphragmatic recess of the pleural cavity (like the spleen). Posteriorly, they lie in contact with quadratus lumborum and the subcostal, iliohypogastric and ilioinguinal nerves (Fig. 3.36.2, p. 96). The right kidney is posterior to the liver, duodenum and ascending colon, while the left lies behind the stomach, spleen, pancreas, jejunum and descending colon. The hilum lies approximately in the transpyloric plane (L1) and is continuous internally with the renal pelvis.

Ureter

The ureter is a narrow muscular duct that propels urine by peristalsis from the hilum of the kidney to the bladder. The duct is approximately 25 cm long and is lined by transitional epithelium. The renal pelvis is the superior expanded end of the ureter; it receives urine from the tubular system of the kidney (Fig. 3.35.2) and is subject to significant anatomical variation. Urine drains from the renal papillae into minor and major calyces, which are continuous with the renal pelvis (Fig. 3.35.2).

The abdominal course of the ureter is retroperitoneal. It lies on the medial border of psoas major, crossing the tips of the transverse processes of the lumbar vertebrae and the bifurcation of the common iliac artery at the sacroiliac joint (Fig. 3.35.3). It runs on the lateral wall of the pelvis before piercing the bladder

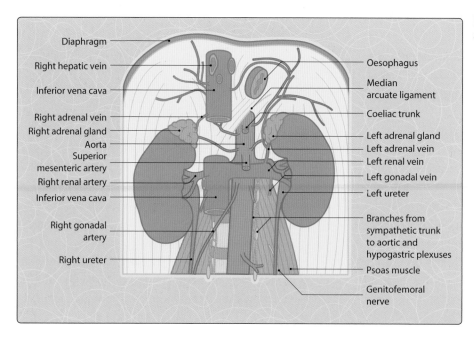

Fig. 3.35.1 Anterior view of the kidneys, adrenal glands and related vessels.

Diaphragm

Right hepatic vein

Inferior vena cava

Right adrenal vein
Right adrenal gland
Aorta
Superior mesenteric artery
Right renal artery
Inferior vena cava

Right gonadal artery

Right ureter

Oesophagus

Median arcuate ligament

Coeliac trunk

Left adrenal gland
Left adrenal vein
Left renal vein
Left gonadal vein
Left ureter

Branches from sympathetic trunk to aortic and hypogastric plexuses

Psoas muscle

Genitofemoral nerve

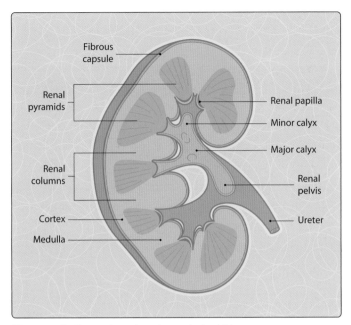

Fig. 3.35.2 Coronal section through the kidney.

at the level of the ischial spine. These bony landmarks can be visualized on a radiograph of the abdomen. The course through the bladder wall (intravesical) is oblique, about 2 cm long and creates a valve-like arrangement, which prevents reflux of urine into the ureters (p. 103).

Adrenal glands

The adrenals are important endocrine glands that lie like caps on the upper poles of the kidneys (Fig. 3.35.1). They consist of an outer cortex, which secretes steroid hormones, and inner medulla, which consists of modified *neurons*; these release adrenaline (epinephrine) and noradrenaline (norepinephrine) in response to sympathetic stimulation. The right suprarenal gland is relatively inaccessible, lying posterior to inferior vena cava and liver. The left is related to the spleen, stomach, pancreas and left crus of the diaphragm.

Blood supply of the kidneys, ureters and adrenal glands

Renal arteries receive about 25% of the cardiac output via direct lateral branches of the abdominal aorta at the level of L1. The right renal artery is long and passes posterior to the inferior vena cava. Each renal artery divides into five segmental branches at the hilum that do not anastomose within the kidney (they are **end arteries**; see p. 9).

The renal vein forms from segmental veins anterior to the renal pelvis and artery at the hilum. The left vein is longer than the right; it receives the left gonadal veins and passes anterior to the abdominal aorta before draining to the inferior vena cava.

The suprarenal glands have a rich blood supply comprising the:

- superior suprarenal arteries: branches of the inferior phrenic arteries (branches of the coeliac trunk)
- middle suprarenal arteries: direct from the abdominal aorta
- inferior suprarenal arteries: from the renal arteries.

The right suprarenal vein drains to the inferior vena cava and the left to the left renal vein.

The ureters receive blood from lumbar segmental arteries, renal and gonadal arteries, the aorta and branches of the internal iliac and inferior vesical arteries.

Lymphatic drainage

Lymph vessels of the kidney and adrenals drain from the hilum to para-aortic nodes.

 URETERIC CALCULI/KIDNEY STONES

Kidney stones may cause obstruction of urinary flow and distension of the ureter. They present as very severe rhythmic pain (renal colic) from loin to groin. There may also be haematuria (blood in the urine). There are three sites of constriction where kidney stones are likely to get stuck:
- junction of the pelvis with the ureter
- as the ureter crosses the pelvic brim
- as the ureter passes through the bladder wall (narrowest).
Stones can sometimes be disrupted by lithotripsy, where they are bombarded with ultrasound radiation.

36. Posterior abdominal wall

Questions
- Which branches of the lumbar plexus supply abdominal structures?
- Which division of the autonomic nervous system slows peristalsis of the gut tube?
- What is the origin of the parasympathetic supply of the descending colon?

Bones

The posterior wall is supported by the bodies of the five lumbar vertebrae, with their intervertebral discs, the sacrum and ilium.

Muscles

There are three prevertebral muscles on each side. They act as a group to flex the vertebral column (Fig. 3.36.1).

- Laterally **quadratus lumborum** arises from the posterior part of the iliac crest and attaches superiorly to the 12th rib. It can sometimes assist inspiration and laterally flexes the vertebral column. It is enclosed in **thoracolumbar fascia,** which extends laterally and gives attachment to the muscles of the anterior abdominal wall.
- Medially **psoas major** and **minor** arise from lumbar vertebrae L1–L4 and attach distally with the iliacus to the lesser trochanter of the femur. They flex the trunk on the lower limb. Abscesses can develop in the abdominal part of the muscle sheath and spread inferiorly to appear below the inguinal ligament.

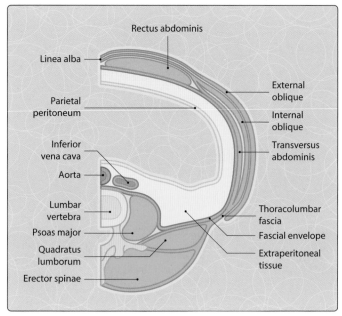

Fig. 3.36.1 Transverse section of the posterior abdominal wall.

Posterior part of the diaphragm

Review the thoracic description of the diaphragm (Figs 3.23.1 and 3.23.2). From the abdominal aspect, the right and left **crura** arise from the lumbar vertebrae and blend with the muscular domes of the diaphragm. The right crus arises from L1–L3 vertebrae, whereas the left is attached to L1 and L2. The fibres of the right crus loop around the terminal part of the oesophagus. The **median arcuate ligament** arches between the two crura to

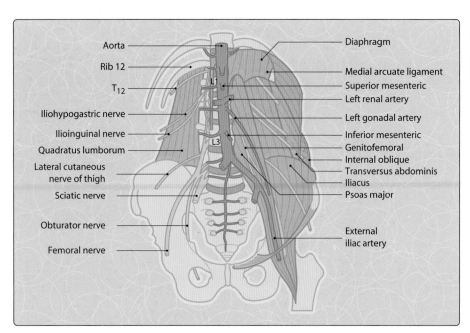

Fig. 3.36.2 Anterior view of the posterior abdominal wall. On the right of the figure, psoas major is intact and on the left, psoas major and the common iliac artery have been removed to show the lumbar plexus.

form the anterior border of the aortic hiatus (see Fig. 3.23.1). On either side, there are thickenings in the fascia over psoas and quadratus lumborum, which form the **medial** and **lateral arcuate ligaments**.

A layer of fascia covers the muscles forming the anterior and posterior abdominal walls (Fig. 3.36.1). It separates the parietal peritoneum from the muscles and is named according to the muscle that it overlies (e.g. transversalis fascia anteriorly and psoas fascia posteriorly).

Blood vessels
See Fig. 3.35.1.

Nerves
The **subcostal** nerve is the ventral ramus of T_{12}. It passes obliquely across quadratus lumborum to supply the muscles and skin of the anterior abdominal wall. The **lumbar plexus** forms from ventral rami of L_1–L_4 within the psoas muscle (Fig. 3.36.2 and Fig. 3.44.1). Table 3.36.1 shows the relation of nerves to the psoas.

Autonomic nerves and plexuses
In the thorax, there are complex interconnected plexuses of sympathetic and parasympathetic fibres at the bifurcation of the trachea (pulmonary, cardiac and oesophageal plexuses). There are similar arrangements in the abdomen. The preaortic plexuses surround the abdominal aorta and its anterior branches to form the **coeliac**, **superior mesenteric** and **inferior mesenteric plexuses**. Sympathetic fibres synapse in prevertebral ganglia within the plexuses and postganglionic fibres are distributed on blood vessels. Parasympathetic fibres synapse in the walls of the viscera. The superior and inferior **hypogastric plexuses** lie at the bifurcation of the aorta and they supply the pelvic organs.

Parasympathetic nerves
The abdominal parasympathetic nerves *only* supply the gut tube and its derivatives. The anterior and posterior vagal trunks supply the gut as far as the splenic flexure. Parasympathetic preganglionic fibres are also carried in spinal nerves S_2–S_4 and form the **pelvic splanchnic nerves**, forming the inferior hypogastric plexus to sigmoid colon, rectum and pelvic organs.

Sympathetic nerves
The sympathetic trunks pass behind the medial arcuate ligaments of the diaphragm to enter the abdomen. However, the main sympathetic supply to the abdominal viscera is the greater, lesser and least splanchnic nerves, which arise from the *thoracic* sympathetic trunk. These nerves pierce the corresponding crus of the diaphragm to synapse in the ganglia of the preaortic plexuses. **Lumbar splanchnic nerves** arise from the lumbar region of the sympathetic trunk and synapse in the inferior mesenteric and superior hypogastric plexuses. Postganglionic fibres from the inferior mesenteric plexus supply the distal part of the colon. Note that there are sympathetic sensory as well as motor fibres; they register visceral sensation such as distension. The sympathetic chain ends in the pelvis as the ganglion impar.

Table 3.36.1 NERVES OF THE PSOAS

Nerve	Relationship to psoas	Supplies
Femoral nerve (L_2, L_3, L_4)	Emerges from the lateral border	Extensor compartment of the thigh
Lateral cutaneous nerve of the thigh (L_2, L_3)	Emerges from the lateral border	Lateral skin
Ilioinguinal (L_1)	Emerges from the lateral border	Inferior part of lower abdominal wall and anterior genital skin
Iliohypogastric (L_1)		Anterior part of the genitals and cremaster muscle
Genitofemoral (L_1, L_2)	Anterior	Anterior part of the genitals and cremaster muscle
Obturator (L_2, L_3, L_4)	Medial	Adductors of the thigh
Lumbosacral trunk	Medial	Contributes to the sacral plexus

37. Pelvis

Questions
- Which ligaments stabilize the pelvic girdle?
- What structures form the walls and floor of the pelvis?
- How can pelvic malignancy spread to the lumbar vertebral bodies?

Pelvic walls

Review the hip bones and sacrum that form the pelvic girdle (Fig. 3.37.1A and p. 107). The pubic bones meet at the **pubic symphysis,** which is a secondary cartilagenous joint allowing little movement. The sacroiliac joints are stabilized by the **sacrotuberous** and **sacrospinous ligaments** together with the **iliolumbar** and **sacroiliac ligaments** (Fig. 3.37.1B).

The **pelvic brim** (or **inlet**) consists of the sacral promontory (Fig. 3.37.1B), arcuate lines of the ilium and the pubic symphysis. The **outlet** is bounded by the coccyx, sacrotuberous ligaments, ischial tuberosities and pubic arch. The overall size of the pelvic cavity and the dimensions of the inlet and outlet are larger in women (to accommodate fetal development and childbirth).

The side wall of the pelvis is formed by the hip bone and the obturator internus muscle. It is attached to the internal surface of the obturator membrane. The posterior wall is formed by the sacrum and the piriformis muscle.

Pelvic floor/diaphragm

Levator ani and coccygeus are the muscles that form a *funnel-shaped diaphragm* separating the pelvic cavity from the perineum below (Fig. 3.37.2A,B). It is pierced by the urethra and rectum and by the vagina. It supports the pelvic organs and forms part of the anal and urinary sphincters. The most inferior part of the funnel lies between the anus and the vagina/scrotum, where a condensation of fibromuscular tissue forms the important **perineal body** (Fig. 3.37.2B,C). The perineal body is fused to levator ani and the external anal sphincter.

Pelvic cavity and peritoneum

The pelvic part of the peritoneal cavity is limited by the walls of the pelvis with the rectum behind and the bladder and anterior abdominal wall in front.

The pelvic fascia is continuous with the fascial lining of the abdominal cavity and the perineum. It forms a strong membrane over the obturator externus and piriformis muscles and condenses to form the puboprostatic and pubovesical ligaments, which support the bladder.

Folds of the peritoneum lining the pelvis form ligaments and recesses (see Figs 3.39.1 for the male and 3.40.1 for the female). To understand the **broad ligament,** think of the uterus and the uterine tubes growing up from below into the peritoneal cavity. The broad ligament is the double layer of peritoneum that dangles between the tubes and the floor and lateral walls of the pelvis. It encloses the uterine tubes, uterine and ovarian vessels, nerves and lymphatics. The ureters pass under the base of the broad ligament close to the lateral fornix of the vagina to reach the bladder.

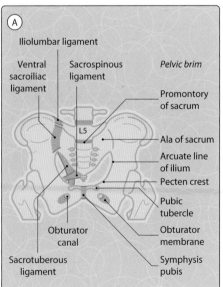
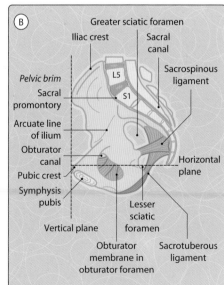
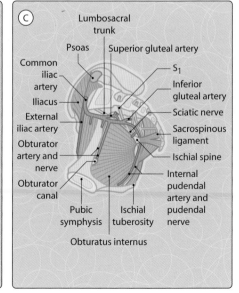

Fig. 3.37.1 The pelvis. (A) Anterior view of the bony pelvis; (B) median sagittal section showing internal surface; (C) median sagittal section showing sacral plexus and branches of the internal iliac artery on the lateral wall.

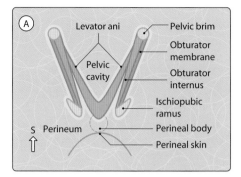

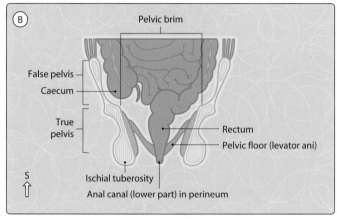

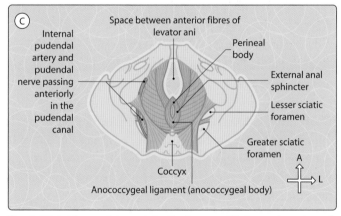

Fig. 3.37.2 Views of the pelvic diaphragm. (A) Coronal section of the pelvis to show the attachment of the pelvic diaphragm to the obturator internus; (B) coronal section of the pelvis more posteriorly to show the rectum passing through the pelvic diaphragm; (C) pelvic diaphragm from below.

The peritoneal recess between the uterus and rectum is the **rectouterine pouch of Douglas** (Fig. 3.40.2) and normally contains coils of ilium. Notice the position of the posterior fornix of the vagina and the pouch of Douglas. It may be used to gain access to the peritoneal cavity.

Blood supply

The supply to the pelvis arises primarily from the internal iliac arteries (p. 110). On the lateral wall of the pelvis, the **anterior division** of the internal iliac gives a number of branches:

- superior and inferior vesical arteries
- middle rectal artery, which anastomoses with the rectal branches of the inferior mesenteric (the equivalent veins are a site of portosystemic anastomosis; p. 85)
- reproductive organs (except the ovary and testis, which are supplied directly from the aorta)
- internal pudendal artery to the perineum (p. 100)
- obturator artery (p. 110)
- inferior gluteal (p. 110).

The **posterior division** gives the superior gluteal artery, which supplies the gluteal muscles, and branches that supply the body wall and spinal cord (iliolumbar and lateral sacral arteries).

The pelvic viscera drain into veins that unite to form the internal iliac veins (except the gonadal veins). The pelvic veins also have connections to the vertebral venous plexus, which accounts for the haematogenous spread of pelvic cancer to lumbar vertebral bodies (e.g. prostate cancer).

THE PERINEAL BODY AND EPISIOTOMY

The peroneal body is more mobile in women as the position of the vagina means that it lacks the support of the perineal membranes. A peroneal tear that damages the perineal body may result in double incontinence and prolapse of pelvic organs. Such tears can occur during delivery of a baby. Episiotomy is an incision made obliquely, avoiding the perineal body, to enlarge the vaginal opening during childbirth. Local anaesthetic injected through the vaginal wall around the ischial spine infiltrates and blocks the pudendal nerve (p. 100).

38. Perineum

Questions
- What is the lymphatic drainage of the lower part of the anal canal?
- What is the nerve supply of the perineum?

The perineum is the diamond-shaped area between the thighs separated from the peritoneal cavity by the pelvic diaphragm. All perineal structures are supplied by the pudendal nerve (S_2–S_4) and internal pudendal artery. It is usually divided into two regions, posterior (anal) and anterior (urogenital) (Fig. 3.38.1).

Anal triangle

The posterior triangle is the same in both sexes and contains the anal canal lying between the ischioanal fossae.

The **anal canal** is 4 cm long and passes down and backwards from the rectum within the perineum (see also p. 102). The **anorectal junction** is pulled abruptly forwards by the puborectalis component of levator ani. Its anatomy is complicated because it marks the boundary between the inside and outside of the body (Fig. 3.38.2). Around its midpoint internally is the pectinate or white line, marking a developmental transition between the endoderm of the gut tube and ectoderm of the skin (Table 3.38.1). Piles (haemorrhoids) and abscesses can develop here.

The **internal sphincter** of the anal canal is derived from the inner circular layer of the gut tube (involuntary control). It surrounds the upper three-quarters of the canal and overlaps with the **external sphincter,** which is striated muscle (voluntary control via S_4 and inferior rectal nerve). The external sphincter

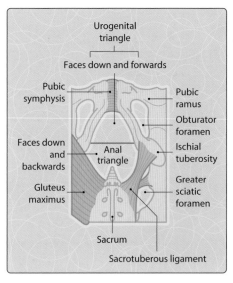

Fig. 3.38.1 Schematic view of the pelvis from below.

blends with fibres of **puborectalis** (part of the levator ani) and can be palpated in a rectal examination as the anorectal ring (Fig. 3.38.2). Damage to the external sphincter or the perineal body can cause anal incontinence.

The **ischioanal fossae** (Fig. 3.38.2) lie to either side of the anal canal below the pelvic floor, between obturator internus and levator ani; inferiorly is perineal skin. The space is fat filled to allow expansion of the anal canal during defaecation. Consequently, abscesses here can enlarge and even spread to the opposite side. The **pudendal canals** conveying the **pudendal nerve,** and **internal pudendal vessels** lie on the lateral walls. The nerve and vessels emerge from the pelvis below piriformis into the gluteal region, crossing the ischial spine before passing back into the pelvis through the lesser sciatic foramen. As they run

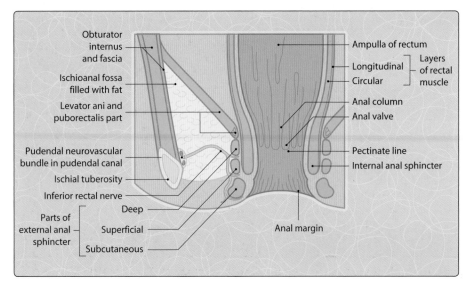

Fig. 3.38.2 Coronal section of the rectum, anal canal and ischioanal fossa.

Table 3.38.1 DIFFERENCES BETWEEN THE UPPER AND LOWER PARTS OF THE ANAL CANAL

	Upper anal canal	Lower anal canal
Epithelium lining	Columnar	Stratified squamous (skin)
Internal features	Anal columns overlying blood vessels; anal valves and sinuses	Puckered skin
Arterial supply	Superior rectal from the inferior mesenteric; middle rectal from the internal iliac	Inferior rectal from the internal pudendal
Venous drainage	Superior rectal vein drains to the portal vein	Internal pudendal veins
Lymphatic drainage	Internal iliac nodes drain to preaortic nodes	Superficial inguinal nodes
Pain sensation	Insensitive (autonomic)	Sensitive (inferior rectal nerve)

forward in the pudendal canal towards the deep perineal space, they divide to form inferior rectal nerves (S_3, S_4), which pass medially to supply levator ani, anal sphincters, anal canal and skin, the dorsal nerve of the clitoris or penis and the perineal nerve.

Urogenital triangle

The urogenital triangle is the region between the pubic rami and perineal body behind. Spanning the space and *inferior* to the *pelvic* diaphragm is the **urogenital diaphragm**, comprising

- superior layer of fascia
- sheet of *voluntary* perineal muscle that forms the external urinary sphincter (anteriorly sphincter urethrae and posteriorly deep transverse perineal muscles)
- the **perineal membrane**, a horizontal fibrous sheet (denser in males) that separates the superficial and deep perineal spaces.

The diaphragm is pierced by the urethra (and the vagina in women).

Male

The **deep perineal space** contains the sphincter urethrae, the membranous part of the urethra, bulbourethral (Cowper's) glands, the dorsal nerves of the penis and internal pudendal vessels (Fig. 3.38.3). The **superficial space** contains the root of the penis, the scrotal nerves and blood vessels and three muscles: **superficial transverse perineal** muscle between the perineal body and the ischial ramus; **ischiocavernosus,** covering the crura of the penis (corpus spongiosum); and **bulbospongiosus,** surrounding the bulb of the penis (corpus cavernosum, p. 103).

Female

The **deep perineal space** contains the sphincter urethrae, urethra, dorsal nerves of the clitoris and internal pudendal vessels (Fig. 3.38.3B). The **superficial perineal space** contains labial nerves and blood vessels and the crura of the clitoris, covered by ischiocavernosus muscle. The fibres of bulbospongiosus surround the vestibule and insert into the clitoris.

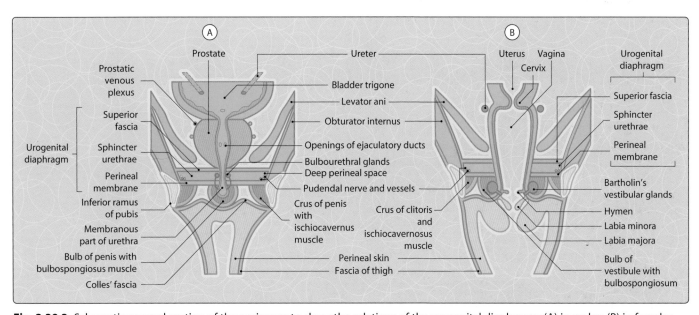

Fig. 3.38.3 Schematic coronal section of the perineum to show the relations of the urogenital diaphragm: (A) in males; (B) in females.

39. Male pelvic viscera and external genitalia

Questions
- What symptoms are associated with prostatic hypertrophy?
- Which part of the urethra is likely to give problems when a catheter is being inserted?
- Where are metastases from prostate cancer likely to occur?

The normal development and function of the organs of the male reproductive system (Fig. 3.39.1) depend on the secretion of testosterone by the testis.

Male genital system

The **ductus (vas) deferens** is a muscular tube running from the tail of the epididymis through the inguinal canal in the spermatic cord (p. 78). It passes posteriorly, crossing the external iliac vessels and looping over the ureter to reach the base of the bladder (Fig. 3.39.2). Here it expands to form the **ampulla** before joining the duct of the seminal vesicle to form the **ejaculatory duct,** which pierces the base of the prostate and opens into the prostatic urethra.

The prostate

Like the seminal vesicles, the **prostate** secretes seminal fluid, which suspends and sustains spermatozoa at ejaculation. The base of the prostate is fixed to the underside of the bladder with its apex supported by the urogenital diaphragm and the anterior fibres of levator ani. The gland is divided into functional zones by thick fibromuscular septa and is surrounded by a capsule and

a layer of pelvic fascia. Most importantly, the prostate *completely* surrounds the proximal (prostatic) urethra. Its **blood supply** arises from the inferior vesical artery. Veins drain to the prostatic venous plexus between the capsule and pelvic fascia via the internal iliac veins to the aorta (so prostatic cancer can spread to vertebrae).

Urethra and penis

Catheterization of the male urethra is a common procedure (e.g. when prostatic hypertrophy leads to urinary obstruction in the elderly). For this reason, you must know the anatomy of the urethra (Fig. 3.39.1B). There are four sections.

1. **Prostatic:** at this point the urethra has a wide U-shaped lumen and is surrounded by the prostate.
2. **Membranous:** pierces the urogenital diaphragm and turns forwards through 90 degrees where there is a slight dilatation (bulb). It can be tricky to pass the catheter around this corner and through the sphincter urethrae.
3. **Spongy:** surrounded by the corpus spongiosum.
4. **Penile:** enclosed within the penis; close to the tip, there is a fold in the lining of the navicular fossa that tends to obstruct the passage of the catheter.

The penis is formally described in its *erect* position as having dorsal and ventral surfaces, so 'normally' its dorsal surface is in front! It is in effect an enlarged clitoris and consists of three cylinders of erectile tissue (Fig. 3.39.3). The **corpus spongiosum** lies in the midline and surrounds the urethra. It is fixed to the urogenital diaphragm by the bulbospongiosus muscle and

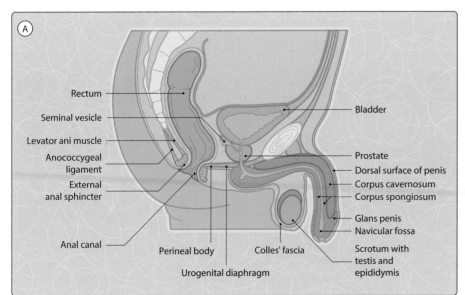

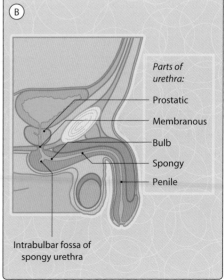

Fig. 3.39.1 Median sagittal sections of the male pelvis (A) and the regions of the male urethra (B).

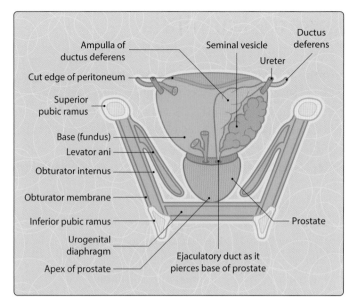

Fig. 3.39.2 Posterior view of the bladder showing the ductus deferens, ampulla and seminal vesicles.

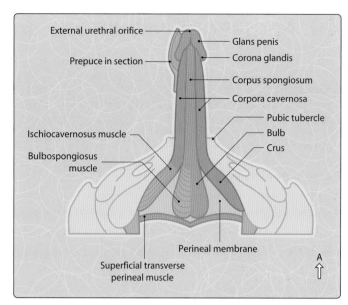

Fig. 3.39.3 Inferior view of the root of the penis.

enlarges distally forming the **glans penis**. The ischiocavernosus muscles attach the **corpora cavernosa** to the inferior pubic rami. They do not contribute to the glans.

Blood is supplied by the pudendal arteries, which then drain to the prostatic venous plexus and internal iliac veins.

To remember the **autonomic nerve supply**, think of point and shoot: parasympathetic (pelvic splanchnic nerves S_2–S_4) controls erection and sympathetic ejaculation!

The **lymphatic drainage** of the external genitalia is to the inguinal nodes (remember that the testis drains to para-aortic nodes). The rest of the perineal structures drain to internal and external iliac nodes.

Other organs of the pelvic cavity

The wall of the **bladder** consists of three layers of smooth muscle fibres (**detrusor muscle**) lined by transitional epithelium. It lies below the level of the peritoneum and rises into the abdomen as it fills, stripping the peritoneum off the anterior abdominal wall for 3–4 cm. Inferiorly in males, the prostate lies between the neck of the bladder and the urogenital diaphragm. The apex of the bladder is directed forwards and attaches to the umbilicus via the **urachus**, an obliterated embryonic connection. The ureters enter the posterolateral angles of the base of the bladder and the urethral orifice opens inferiorly at the neck. The area between these three openings is the **trigone**. The prostate and bladder are fixed anteriorly by the puboprostatic ligaments and posteriorly by the rectovesical septum (fascia).

The **blood supply** of the bladder is via the superior and inferior vesical arteries, which arise from the internal iliac arteries.

The motor **nerve supply** to the detrusor muscle is via parasympathetic pelvic splanchnic nerves arising from S_2–S_4.

The sigmoid colon and rectum and anal canal are described on pages 93 and 100.

 RECTAL EXAMINATION OF THE PROSTATE

It is possible to feel the prostate through the anterior wall of the rectum. Enlargement occurs in benign hypertrophy and in cancer of the prostate. Malignant change usually affects the peripheral zone, while normal age changes occur in the region that surrounds the prostatic urethra, leading to urinary obstruction.

40. Female pelvic viscera and external genitalia

Questions
- Why is ovarian or uterine pain referred to the inner thigh?
- Why are women predisposed to urinary tract infections?

Female genital system

Ovary

The **ovaries** are solid organs with a vascular medulla and cortical tissue that contains numerous follicles each enclosing a single oocyte. After puberty, monthly cycles of follicular development result in **oestrogen** secretion and ovulation, followed by the production of **progesterone** and, in the absence of pregnancy, **menstruation**. The secretion of hormones ceases at the menopause.

Broad ligament

The ovaries lie close to the lateral walls of the pelvis attached to the posterosuperior surface of the **broad ligament** by the mesovarium (Fig. 3.40.1 and p. 98). They lie close to the course of the obturator nerve, and ovarian disease (and even uterine problems) may present as pain on the inside of the thigh. Like the testes, the ovaries develop opposite L1/L2, but their descent is interrupted by the broad ligament. The female equivalent to the gubernaculum (p. 78) is divided into two, the **ligament of the ovary** and the **round ligament of the uterus**. The first links the ovaries to the uterus and the second runs from the uterus to the labia majora (homologous to the scrotum) via the inguinal canal. The round ligament is small and not associated with inguinal herniae.

Uterine tubes, uterus, vagina and cervix

The uterus and uterine tubes (**Fallopian tubes**) lie inferior to the pelvic peritoneum (Fig. 3.40.2). The uterine tubes are extensions from the upper lateral corners of the uterus lying in the upper edge of the broad ligament. The ciliated epithelial lining transports sperm and oocytes and the developing embryo after fertilization.

There are four regions:

- **infundibulum:** the open end that communicates with the peritoneal cavity; at ovulation the oocyte is swept up by the fimbria and slowly transported to the uterus
- **ampulla:** where fertilization normally occurs
- **isthmus:** the longest part
- **intramural:** passes through the uterine wall.

The uterus has a thick muscular wall (**myometrium**) and a specialized lining (**endometrium**). The lumen is continuous with the uterine tubes superiorly and with the cervix inferiorly.

During the menstrual cycle, the endometrium undergoes dramatic changes in response to ovarian steroids and during early pregnancy it supports the development of the embryo. The uterus consists of the **fundus,** between the openings of the uterine tubes, the **body** and the **cervix**. It narrows inferiorly to the **internal os** of the **cervix,** which opens via the **cervical canal** into the vagina at the **external os.** The cervix is largely composed of tough collagenous material lined by a mucus-secreting simple columnar epithelium. The transition zone at the external os between the columnar epithelium of the cervical canal and the stratified squamous epithelium of the vagina is prone to malignant change and is monitored by **cervical smears**.

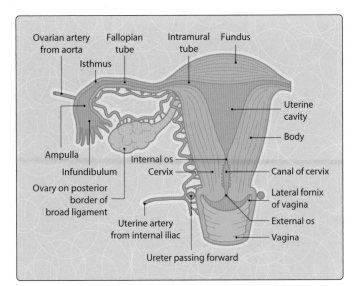

Fig. 3.40.1 Coronal section of the female pelvis and perineum.

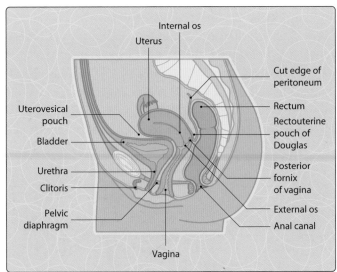

Fig. 3.40.2 Sagittal section of the female pelvis.

The **vagina** has muscular walls lined by stratified squamous epithelium and so this is the site of a squamocolumnar junction (others are the anal canal and gastro-oesophageal junction). The vagina angles up and backwards and the cervix projects into the anterior wall of the vagina forming recesses (the vaginal fornices). The **posterior fornix** gives surgical access to the peritoneal cavity and the **lateral fornices** are very closely related to the ureters on either side (Fig. 3.40.1).

Position and support

In most women the uterus is tilted forward on the backward sloping vagina (**anteverted**). It also is bent forwards on the cervix (**anteflexed**). This means that the uterus flops forwards over the bladder creating a narrow **uterovesical pouch** and a wider **rectouterine pouch** behind. The rectouterine pouch contains coils of ilium and is related to the posterior fornix of the vagina (Fig. 3.40.2).

Pregnancy and childbirth cause massive stresses in the uterus and surrounding tissues and so the mechanical support of the uterus is important.

- pelvic diaphragm acts as a sling for the cervix and vagina.
- ligaments: thickenings of fascia on the upper surface of the diaphragm
  —cardinal: transverse cervical ligaments suspend the cervix from the lateral walls of the pelvis
  —uterosacral: pass backwards from the cervix and vagina to the fascia overlying the sacroiliac joints
  —pubocervical: from the cervix (prostate in males) to the pubic symphysis
  —pubovesical: from the bladder to the pubic symphysis.

Blood and lymphatic systems

The **ovarian artery** (from aorta) supplies the uterine tubes and fundus, it anastomoses with the uterine and vaginal arteries (from internal iliac), which supply the uterus, cervix and vagina.

Veins run in the broad ligament to the internal iliac veins.

Lymphatic drainage of the lower vagina is to the superficial inguinal nodes. The upper vagina, cervix and lower uterine body drain to the internal iliac nodes and the upper body, fundus tubes and ovaries to the para-aortic nodes.

External genitalia

The **vulva** is the name given to the external genitalia (Figs 3.40.3 and 3.40.4). The skin of the **labia majora** is equivalent to scrotal skin; the **clitoris and labia minora** are equivalent to the penis (remember, however, that the urethra *does not* open on the clitoris). The **urethra** is short (3–4 cm) and this predisposes women to ascending urinary tract infections. The urethral meatus lies between the clitoris and the vagina. The **vagina** opens into the vestibule. The hymen is a remnant of the membrane that closes the vagina during embryonic development.

Other organs of the pelvic cavity

In women, the **bladder** rests directly on the pelvic diaphragm (in men the prostate intervenes). As the **ureters** pass forward to enter the base of the bladder, they lie between the lateral vaginal fornices and the uterine arteries. The sigmoid colon, rectum and anal canal are described on pp. 92 and 93.

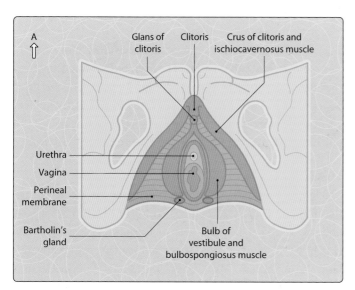

Fig. 3.40.3 Perineal membrane and clitoris from below.

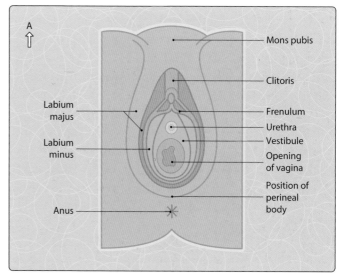

Fig. 3.40.4 Female external genitalia.

41. Development and bones

Questions
- Why are the joints of the lower limb more stable than those of the upper limb?
- Does the line of gravity pass in front of the hip joint?
- Which bones make up the knee joint?

Embryonic development

A generally important point is that the lower limbs undergo medial rotation during development, with the following consequences:

- extensors of the knee lie on the *front* of the thigh while flexors lie *behind* (the opposite arrangement to that in the arm)
- the knee points forwards (elbow points backwards)
- extensors of the toes lie in the anterior compartment and flexors lie in the posterior compartment of the leg (the opposite arrangement to that in the forearm)
- the dorsum of the foot is anterior (dorsum of the hand is posterior)
- the big toe is medial (the thumb is lateral)
- dermatomes spiral round the limb.

Joints

The arrangement of joints in the lower limb is similar to the upper limb. Proximally, like the shoulder, the hip is a ball and socket joint that allows movements in all three planes. The knee is a hinge joint like the elbow and distally the complex articulations of the ankle and subtalar joints allow a range of movement similar to the wrist. There is no equivalent movement in the lower limb to pronation and supination in the upper limb.

The hip, knee and ankle joints carry the entire body weight. They are relatively stable because they must resist the effects of gravity as well as transmitting the forces generated by the powerful muscles of the lower limb (Fig. 3.41.1). The line of gravity passing through the joints influences the position and strength of the ligaments that support them (Fig. 3.41.2). For example, the ligaments of the hip joint are stronger anteriorly to prevent the extension of the joint that tends to occur under gravity.

Hip

The pelvic girdle is a complete bony ring that firmly attaches the lower limbs to the spine (Fig. 3.41.3). It consists of the two hip bones and the sacrum. Each hip bone develops from three bones, the **ilium**, **pubis** and **ischium.** Anteriorly, the two pubic bones articulate at the **pubic symphysis**; posteriorly, the ilium on each

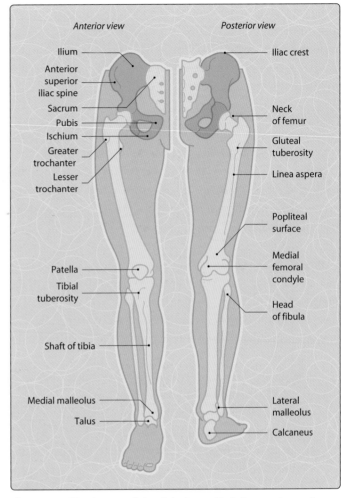

Fig. 3.41.1 The bones of the right lower limb in anterior and posterior view.

side articulates with the sacrum at the **sacroiliac joints** and we sit on our **ischial tuberosities**. The **acetabulum** is a deep bony socket on the outer surface of the hip bone where the three bones meet and where the head of the femur articulates to form a ball and socket joint. The anterior superior iliac spine (ASIS), pubic tubercle and the iliac crest are important bony landmarks.

Thigh

The femoral head is large and fits snugly into the acetabulum at the hip joint. The head is attached to the shaft by a narrow, oblique neck that is vulnerable to fractures, especially in the elderly. At the junction of the neck and shaft are the **greater** and **lesser trochanters**. Anteriorly, the shaft is smooth, but posteriorly there is a pronounced ridge (**linea aspera**) for the attachment of muscles. Distally, there are two massive **condyles** that articulate with the tibia and are separated by the intercondylar notch. The lateral condyle is more prominent

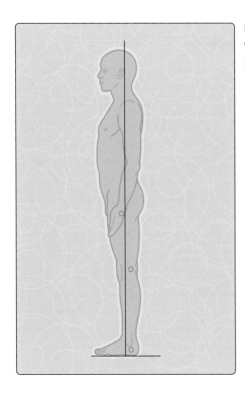

Fig. 3.41.2 The line of gravity as it passes through the lower limb.

the **common fibular nerve** (sometimes common peroneal nerve). Fractures of the fibula may cause damage to the nerve.

Foot

See p. 126.

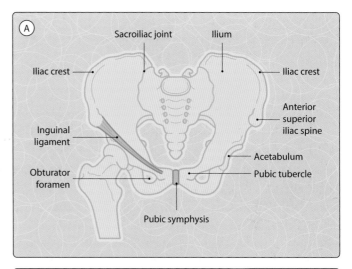

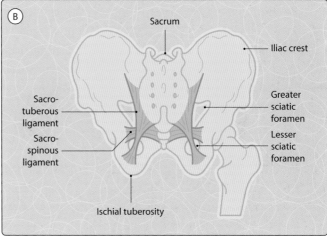

Fig. 3.41.3 The bony pelvis and associated ligaments. (A) Anterior view with inguinal ligament; (B) posterior view.

anteriorly and helps to prevent lateral dislocation of the patella. The **patella** is a triangular, sesamoid bone embedded in the tendon of the quadriceps muscle as it passes anterior to the knee joint. It articulates with both femoral condyles at the knee joint.

In the anatomical position, the distance between your hip joint is greater than the distance between your knee joints and because of this the femur lies at an angle in the thigh. When the quadriceps muscle contracts, it pulls the patella laterally. This means that there is a tendency for the patella to dislocate laterally. This is compensated by two mechanisms. First, the lateral condyle of the femur projects anteriorly forming a bony buttress and, second, the lowest fibres of vastus medialis insert on the medial border of the patella and act to prevent any lateral movement.

Leg

The expanded **medial** and **lateral condyles** of the **tibia** articulate with the condyles of the femur. Anteriorly the **tibial tuberosity** is the point of attachment of the **ligamentum patellae**. The shaft of the tibia (shin) is subcutaneous and trauma can result in an open fracture. The skin over the tibia has a poor blood supply and may be slow to heal. At the distal end of the tibia, the **medial malleolus** forms the medial articular surface of the ankle joint.

Proximally the **fibula** articulates with the lateral tibial condyle but takes no part in the knee joint; distally, the **lateral malleolus** forms the lateral surface of the ankle joint. It is a narrow bone with a palpable head and a narrow neck that is closely related to

 COMMON FRACTURES OF THE LOWER LIMB

- The neck is the weakest part of the femur and fractures may result in avascular necrosis of the head.
- The neck of the fibula is vulnerable to traumatic injury (pedestrians hit by a car bumper). The common fibular nerve lies in contact with the neck and may also be damaged, causing foot drop (p. 123).
- Pott's fracture of the medial malleolus and fibula.

42. Fascia lata, veins and lymphatic drainage

Questions

- Where does the great saphenous vein lie at the ankle?
- What process normally assists venous return from the lower limb?
- What is the lymphatic drainage of the testes?

Fascia lata

The fascia lata is a dense layer of tough inelastic deep fascia that surrounds the leg like a stocking (Fig. 3.42.1). It is attached to the pelvis and ligaments at the root of the limb. At the knee, it attaches to the femur and tibia and is thickened to form the popliteal fascia at the back of the knee. On the lateral side, the fascia lata is thickened to form the **iliotibial tract**, which attaches three-quarters of the fibres of gluteus maximus and tensor fascia lata muscles to the lateral tibial condyle (it helps to stabilize and extend the hip and knee joints). Intermuscular septa attached to the linea aspera of the femur divide the thigh into three compartments (Fig. 3.42.2). Muscles in a compartment share a common function and nerve supply. Haemorrhage within a compartment may cause a rise in pressure that initially may restrict the venous drainage then the arterial supply; nerve and tissue damage may follow. This is **compartment syndrome** and may require surgical intervention.

Veins

Venous blood in the lower limbs must be carried against the force of gravity back to the heart (Fig. 3.42.3; see p. 122). **Superficial veins** lie beneath the skin in the superficial fascia and **deep veins** (or **venae comitantes**) accompany arteries that lie between the muscles within a compartment.

The course of the superficial **great saphenous vein** is constant and important. It arises on the dorsum of the foot and lies anterior to the medial malleolus, where it is used for venepuncture. It travels upwards on the medial side of the leg, knee and thigh before passing through the saphenous opening in fascia lata to empty into the femoral vein. The **small saphenous vein** also begins on the dorsum of the foot but travels behind the lateral malleolus and up the back of the calf before draining into the **popliteal vein** (Fig. 3.42.3). Both superficial veins may be used as grafts in coronary artery bypass surgery.

The **deep veins** in the calf are the veins referred to in 'deep vein thrombosis' (DVT). They join to form the popliteal vein, which lies close to the artery behind the knee and continues as the femoral vein. The superficial and deep veins are connected through a series of **perforating veins** (Fig. 3.42.4).

Lymphatics

All lymph vessels from the superficial parts of the limb drain to the **superficial inguinal nodes**:

- the **vertical group** lies close to the terminal part of the great saphenous vein; they drain most of the limb
- the **horizontal group** lies just below the inguinal ligament; laterally they drain the lower part of the abdominal wall and buttocks and medially they drain the external genitals and lower part of the anal canal. It is significant that, although the scrotum drains to the inguinal nodes, the testes drain directly to aortic nodes in the abdomen (p. 79).

The superficial nodes drain to two or three deep nodes that lie close to the femoral vein and femoral canal. Efferent vessels pass via the external iliac and abdominal nodes to the thoracic duct.

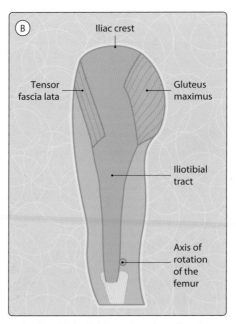

Fig. 3.42.1 Fascia lata and associated structures in the thigh. (A) Anterior view showing inguinal lymph nodes; (B) lateral view showing the iliotibial tract.

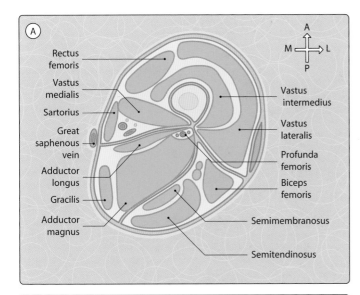

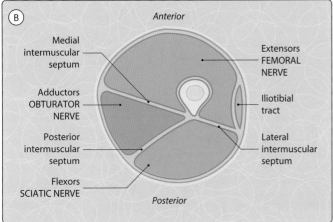

Fig. 3.42.2 Fasia lata and associated structures in the thigh. (A) Anterior view shows the course of the great saphenous vein and the arrangement of the inguinal lymph nodes; (B) lateral view shows the insertion of the iliotibial tract.

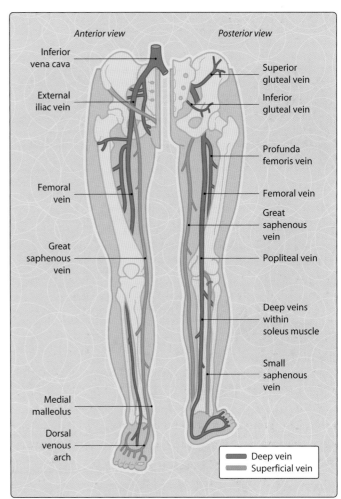

Fig. 3.42.3 The major veins of the lower limb.

VARICOSE VEINS

The weight of the column of blood in the veins of the legs results in increased hydrostatic pressure in those vessels and pooling of venous blood. The perforating veins have one-way valves to ensure flow only from the superficial to the deep veins. Contraction of the calf muscles squeezes the veins, forcing blood up towards the trunk (**calf muscle pump**). If the valves are damaged, blood accumulates in the superficial veins, leading to varicose veins.

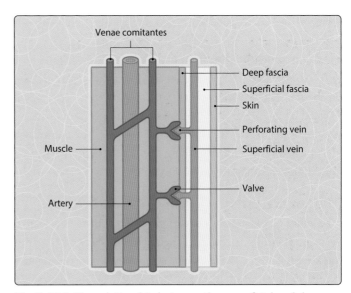

Fig. 3.42.4 The relationship between the superficial and deep veins in the lower limb. Blood normally passes from superficial to deep veins via the perforating veins.

43. Arteries

Questions
- What is the surface marking of the femoral artery as it enters the thigh?
- Which artery supplies most of the muscles of the thigh?
- At what point is the femoral artery in contact with the femur?

The **common iliac artery** divides anterior to the sacroiliac joint forming the internal and external iliac arteries (Figs 3.36.2 and 3.37.1C). It is the **external iliac artery** passing inferiorly under the inguinal ligament that supplies virtually the entire lower limb as the **femoral artery**. Before passing beneath the ligament, the external iliac gives the inferior epigastric artery that will anastomose with the superior epigastric artery in the rectus sheath (Fig. 3.26.4).

The **internal iliac artery** supplies most of the viscera of the pelvis and perineum as well as the muscles of the gluteal region and medial compartment of the thigh. At the edge of the greater sciatic foramen, it divides into anterior and posterior divisions. The branches of the **anterior division** supply the pelvic organs and also the muscles of the buttock and thigh via the **inferior gluteal artery**, which passes through the greater sciatic foramen *inferior* to piriformis (Fig. 3.46.1). The **posterior division** gives the superior gluteal artery, which passes into the gluteal region *superior* to the piriformis muscle (Fig. 3.43.2). The gluteal arteries supply the muscles of the region and join with the circumflex femoral arteries to form the cruciate and trochanteric anastomoses around the hip joint.

The **obturator artery** is also a branch of the anterior division of the internal iliac artery (Fig. 3.37.1). Close to its origin, it is crossed by the ureter. It is closely related to the obturator nerve and vein on the lateral pelvic wall before they all pass through the obturator canal into the thigh. The obturator artery supplies the adductor compartment of the thigh.

The femoral artery

The femoral artery is quite superficial and its pulse can be felt as it enters the thigh at the mid-inguinal point between anterior superior iliac spine and the pubic symphysis (Fig. 3.43.1). At this point, it gives small branches to the region: the superficial circumflex iliac, superficial epigastric and superficial pudendal vessels. In the femoral triangle (p. 114), it gives a large, lateral branch, the deep artery of the thigh (**profunda femoris**), which supplies the medial and posterior muscles of the thigh. The upper branches of profunda femoris (medial and lateral

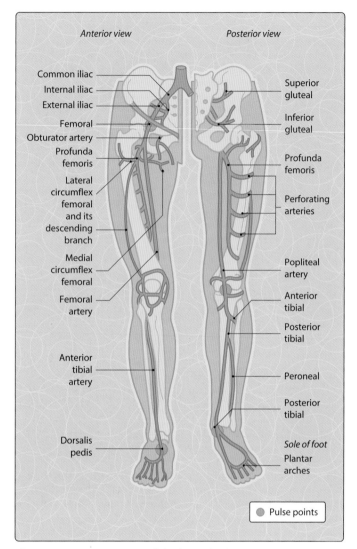

Fig. 3.43.1 Major arteries of the lower limb.

circumflex arteries) encircle the femur at the level of the lesser trochanter, supply the femoral head and contribute to the cruciate and trochanteric anastomoses around the hip joint (p. 119).

The four lower branches of profunda femoris are known as the **perforating branches** because they pierce the insertions of the adductor muscles and the medial intermuscular septum. Since they lie close to the femur, they may be damaged in fractures of the shaft and bleeding from them can be serious.

The continuation of the femoral artery takes a spiral course down the medial side of the thigh under the sartorius muscle (sometimes called the adductor canal; p. 115). It comes into contact with the femur about a hand's breadth above the knee, where it passes through a gap (hiatus) in the adductor magnus muscle and turns behind the knee to lie deep in the **popliteal**

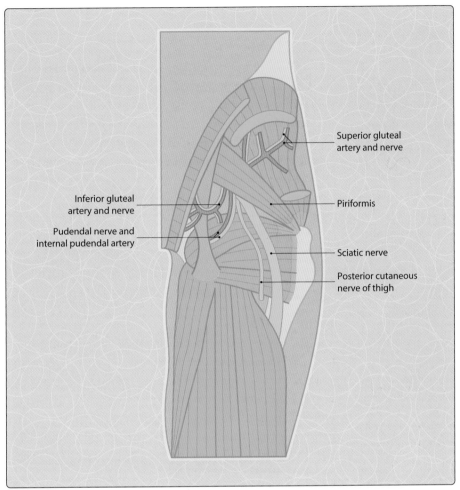

Fig. 3.43.2 Neurovascular structures of the gluteal region. Muscle names are given in Fig. 3.46.1, p. 116.

Superior gluteal artery and nerve

Inferior gluteal artery and nerve

Pudendal nerve and internal pudendal artery

Piriformis

 Sciatic nerve

Posterior cutaneous nerve of thigh

fossa (p. 117). Here it is known as the **popliteal artery** and is covered by a thickening in fascia lata, which makes the popliteal pulse tricky to palpate. About a hand's breadth below the knee it divides into the **anterior** and **posterior tibial arteries**, which supply the leg and foot.

The **anterior tibial** supplies the anterior extensor compartment of the leg and terminates as the **dorsalis pedis artery** on the dorsum of the foot. The larger **posterior tibial artery** passes deeply between the muscles of the calf and gives branches that supply the posterior and lateral compartments of the leg. It passes behind the medial malleolus to supply the sole of the foot through its **medial and lateral plantar arteries**. The lateral plantar artery anastomoses with the dorsalis pedis in a pattern that is similar to the palmar arches of the hand.

ATHEROMA OF THE FEMORAL ARTERY

The femoral artery is prone to arterial disease (atheroma), which causes narrowing and hardening of the arteries. Even mild exercise can cause muscular pain because the reduction in peripheral blood flow causes ischaemia (**intermittent claudication**). For this reason, it is important to understand the pattern of arterial supply and to be able to palpate these pulses:

- **femoral** immediately anterior to the hip joint at the mid-inguinal point
- **popliteal** lies in the popliteal fossa behind the flexed knee and may be difficult to detect
- **dorsalis pedis** is midway between the medial and lateral malleoli in front of the ankle joint, lateral to the tendon of extensor hallucis longus
- **posterior tibial** is under cover of the flexor retinaculum between the calcaneus and the medial malleolus (Figs 3.50.2 and 3.50.4).

44. Nerves

Questions
- Why should you always examine the hip as well as the knee when a patient complains of knee pain?
- Through which space do the branches of the sacral plexus enter the gluteal region?

The lower limb is supplied by the lumbar and sacral plexuses. The general organization is similar to the brachial plexus but they are less vulnerable to damage. Two branches of the lumbar plexus supply the anterior abdominal wall (p. 77); the rest supply the extensor and adductor compartments of the thigh. The sacral plexus supplies all of the rest of the limb.

Lumbar plexus

The lumbar plexus consists of the ventral rami of spinal nerves T_{12}–L_4 (Fig. 3.44.1). It has three lower limb branches.

1. **Lateral cutaneous nerve of thigh** (L_2, L_3) passes under the inguinal ligament where it can become compressed causing paraesthesia in the skin of the thigh.
2. **Obturator nerve** (L_2–L_4) emerges from the pelvis through the obturator foramen (Fig. 3.44.2).
3. **Femoral nerve** (L_2–L_4) is the most lateral structure, passing under the inguinal ligament (Fig. 3.45.2) to supply the extensor compartment of the thigh (Fig. 3.44.3):
   - cutaneous branches supply the anterior skin of the thigh
   - **saphenous nerve,** which is the only branch of the femoral nerve to cross the knee joint (it accompanies the great

saphenous vein in the leg), supplies a strip of skin on the medial side of the leg and foot (dermatome L_4)
- motor branches supply the flexors of the hip (sartorius and iliopsoas); note that these muscles also flex the trunk when the limb is fixed (e.g. when touching the toes)
- motor branches to quadriceps femoris, which is the powerful extensor of the knee
- articular branches supply the hip and knee joints
- motor branches supply the adductor compartment, pectineus, adductor longus, adductor brevis, gracilis and adductor magnus
- cutaneous branches supply the skin on the medial thigh
- articular branches supply both the hip and knee joints.

Sacral plexus

The lumbosacral trunk of the lumbar plexus and the ventral rami of four sacral nerves fuse to form the sacral plexus (L_4, L_5, S_1–S_4, see Fig. 3.44.1) on the posterior wall of the pelvis. The most important pelvic branch is the **pudendal nerve** (S_2–S_4; p. 98). Branches to the lower limb emerge from the pelvis through the greater sciatic foramen deep to gluteus maximus. They include superior gluteal nerve, inferior gluteal nerve, nerve to quadratus femoris (and inferior gamellus), nerve to obturator internus (and superior gamellus), posterior cutaneous nerve of thigh and sciatic nerve (L_4, L_5, S_1–S_3), which is the largest nerve in the body.

The sciatic nerve supplies the flexor compartment of the thigh (Fig. 3.44.4) and its terminal branches supply the limb below the knee (Fig. 3.44.4B,C; see also pp. 123 and 125).

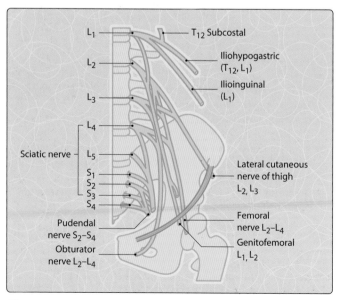

Fig. 3.44.1 Anterior view of the lumbar and sacral plexuses and their branches.

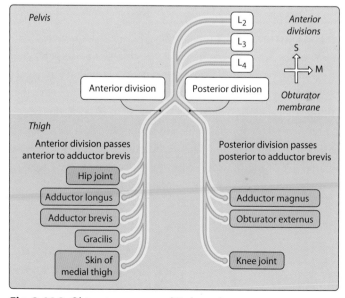

Fig. 3.44.2 Obturator nerve and its branches.

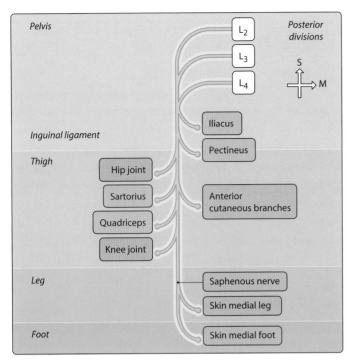

Fig. 3.44.3 Femoral nerve and its branches.

 KNEE AND HIP PAIN

The hip and knee joints receive articular branches from both the femoral and obturator nerves. This double innervation explains why disease of the hip joint often presents as pain in the knee (it is an important example of referred pain).

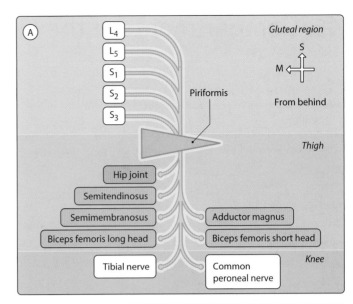

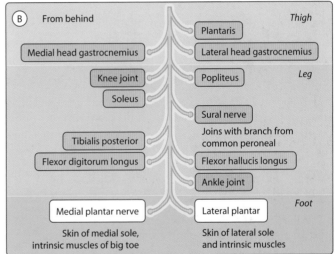

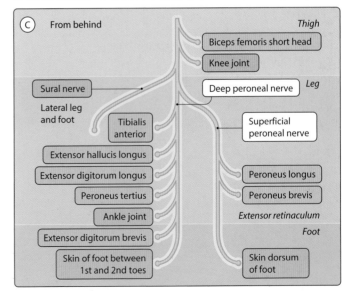

Fig. 3.44.4 The sciatic nerve. (A) supply to posterior compartment of the thigh; (B) tibial nerve and branches; (C) common peroneal nerve and branches.

45. Compartments of the thigh and the femoral triangle

Questions
- What is the nerve supply of the three compartments of the thigh?
- What are the contents of the femoral triangle?
- What is the significance of the femoral canal?

Compartments

The fascia lata extends between the muscles to form three intermuscular septa that attach to the linea aspera of the femur, dividing the thigh into three compartments (Fig. 3.42.2, p. 109).

Anterior (extensor) compartment

The anterior (extensor) compartment contains iliopsoas, sartorius and quadriceps femoris (Fig. 3.45.1). Quadriceps has four heads, rectus femoris, vastus lateralis, vastus medialis and vastus intermedius, which lies deep to the other heads. The tendons of the four heads fuse to form the quadriceps tendon, which inserts into the upper border of the patella and continues inferiorly as the patellar ligament, which inserts on the tibial tuberosity. Quadriceps is a powerful extensor of the knee. The compartment is supplied by the femoral nerve (L_2–L_4) and the branches of the profunda femoris artery.

Medial (adductor) compartment

The medial (adductor) compartment contains pectineus and the adductor longus, adductor brevis and adductor magnus (Fig. 3.42.2B). Note that these muscles adduct and laterally rotate the hip but their everyday action is to *prevent unwanted* abduction and medial rotation (think of Bambi's legs sliding out from under him when he tried to walk on the ice: *that* was unwanted abduction!). The compartment is supplied by the obturator nerve (L_2–L_4) and branches of the obturator and profunda femoris arteries.

Posterior (flexor) compartment

The posterior (flexor) compartment contains the three hamstrings, biceps femoris, semitendinosus and semimembranosus. They extend the hip and flex the knee (Fig. 3.42.2B). The compartment is supplied by the sciatic nerve (L_4, L_5, S_1–S_3) and the perforating branches of the profunda femoris artery.

Femoral triangle

The boundaries of the femoral triangle (Fig. 3.45.2) are:
- superiorly: **inguinal ligament** (the lower edge of the external oblique muscle attached laterally to anterior superior iliac spine and medially to the pubic tubercle)
- laterally: **sartorius**

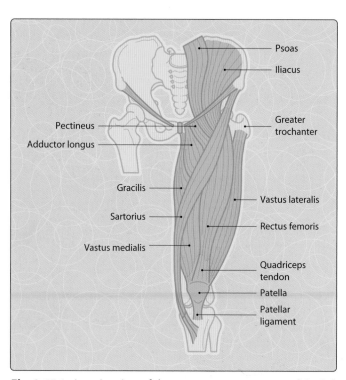

Fig. 3.45.1 Anterior view of the extensor compartment of the left thigh.

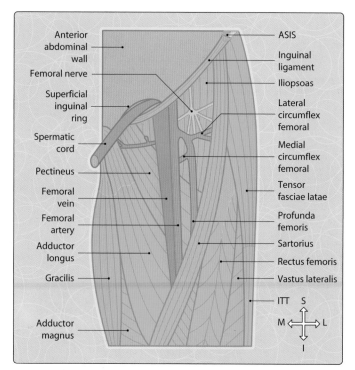

Fig. 3.45.2 Anterior view of the femoral triangle and its contents (left thigh).

- medially: **adductor longus**
- floor, from lateral to medial: **iliopsoas**, **pectineus**, **adductor longus**
- roof: **fascia lata**.

The contents from lateral to medial are:

- **femoral nerve** lateral to the femoral pulse
- **femoral artery** passes posterior to the inguinal ligament at the mid-inguinal point
- **femoral vein** medial to the femoral pulse.

The artery and vein (*not* the nerve) enter the triangle enclosed in the **femoral sheath**, a tube of fascia like a funnel and continuous with the abdominal fascial lining (Fig. 3.45.3). It is divided into three compartments, one each for the artery and vein and the most medial, the **femoral canal**, which is occupied by lymphatics and a single lymph node.

Femoral canal

The femoral canal is a site of potential weakness through which abdominal contents (gut, fat) may herniate into the femoral canal. The abdominal side of the femoral canal is the **femoral ring**, its boundaries are:

- anteriorly: **inguinal ligament**
- medially: **lacunar ligament** (part of the inguinal ligament) the sharp edge may cause strangulation of the hernia
- posteriorly: **superior ramus of the pubis**
- laterally: **femoral vein**.

A femoral hernia becomes obvious when it is large enough to pass from the canal through the saphenous opening in fascia lata, which lies below and lateral to the pubic tubercle (Fig. 3.42.1A). It is more common in women because the female pelvis is wider.

Adductor canal

The femoral vessels leave the apex of the femoral triangle in the adductor canal, which is covered anteriorly by sartorius (hence its alternative name the subsartorial canal). Initially, vastus medialis forms the lateral boundary of the canal and adductor longus forms the medial boundary. Closer to the knee, adductor magnus replaces adductor longus. The femoral vein spirals behind the artery in the canal, so when the vessels pass posteriorly through a gap in adductor magnus (the **adductor hiatus**) to reach the back of the knee, the vein is more superficial than the artery in the popliteal fossa. As it passes through the hiatus, the femoral artery lies in contact with the femur. The nerve to vastus medialis and the saphenous nerve also lie in the adductor canal. The saphenous nerve accompanies the great saphenous vein on the medial side of the leg and supplies skin on the medial side of the leg and foot.

KNEE JERK

Tapping the patellar tendon causes contraction of the quadriceps muscle (knee jerk). It is a test for the femoral nerve and spinal segments L_3 and L_4.

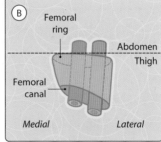

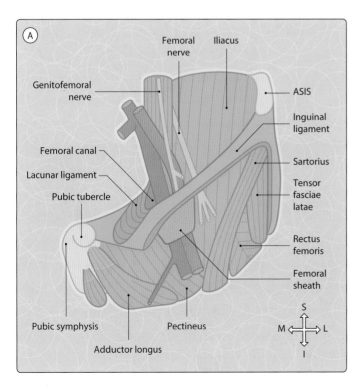

Fig. 3.45.3 The femoral sheath left thigh. (A) Anterior view of the femoral triangle to show the femoral sheath; (B) anterior view to show the position of the femoral canal; (C) lateral view of the fascial layer that forms the femoral sheath.

46. Gluteal region and back of thigh

Questions
- What are the functions of the gluteus maximus, medius and minimis?
- What is the nerve supply of the hamstring muscles?
- Where should you place an intramuscular injection in the buttock and why?

The gluteal region (Fig. 3.46.1) is covered by a thick layer of superficial fascia (commonly known as fat!).

Bony and ligamentous features

Sacrotuberous and **sacrospinous ligaments** (Fig. 3.37.1) convert the sciatic notches of the hip bones into the **greater sciatic** and the **lesser sciatic foramina.** The greater sciatic foramen is the gateway leading from the pelvis to the thigh. The lesser foramen is the gateway from the gluteal region to the perineum (Fig. 3.37.1).

Muscles

Gluteus maximus is a powerful muscle that extends the flexed hip joint (particularly when standing up from a sitting position or walking up stairs).

Gluteus medius and **minimus** muscles are active when one foot is taken off the ground (e.g. when walking). They prevent the pelvis from dipping down on the unsupported side (Fig. 3.46.2). If these muscles are paralysed a patient will walk with a characteristic 'dipping gait' as the pelvis tilts down on the unsupported side. This is known as a positive Trendelenburg test.

The **lateral rotator muscles** of the hip lie on the posterior aspect of the hip joint:

- piriformis
- superior gamellus
- obturator internus
- inferior gamellus
- quadratus femoris.

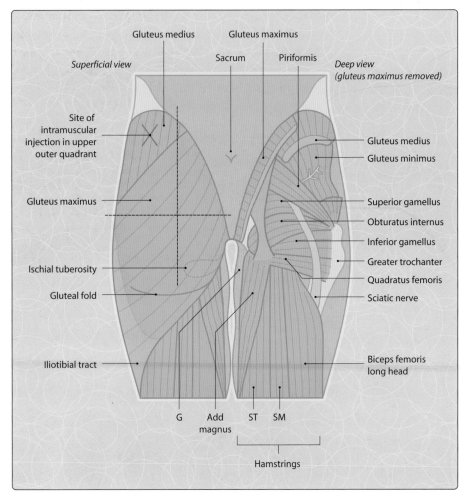

Fig. 3.46.1 Posterior view of the gluteal region. Removal of the gluteus maximus and part of gluteus minimus reveals the relations of the sciatic nerve, and the origin of the hamstring muscles (right).

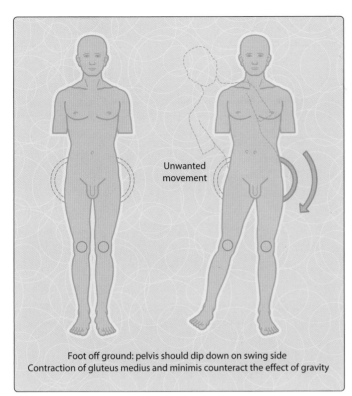

Foot off ground: pelvis should dip down on swing side
Contraction of gluteus medius and minimis counteract the effect of gravity

Fig. 3.46.2 When one foot is raised from the ground, the unsupported pelvis should dip down on that side. Contraction of gluteus medius and minimus counteracts the effects of gravity.

The lateral rotator muscles are equivalent to the rotator cuff muscles of the glenohumeral joint (p. 42); they are not important to the stability of the hip.

Nerves and vessels

The **superior gluteal nerve** (L_4, L_5, S_1) emerges from the greater sciatic foramen *above* piriformis (Fig. 3.43.2); it lies between the gluteus medius and minimis and passes anteriorly accompanied by the superior gluteal artery to supply gluteus medius and minimis and fasciae latae muscles.

Structures that emerge from the greater sciatic foramen *below* piriformis are:

- **inferior gluteal nerve** (L_5, S_1, S_2) is accompanied by the inferior gluteal artery and supplies the gluteus maximus

- **posterior cutaneous nerve of the thigh** (S_1–S_3) supplies the skin of the buttock, external genitalia and the back of the thigh
- **sciatic nerve** (L_4, L_5, S_1, S_2) passes over the lateral rotator muscles posterior to the hip joint before giving muscular branches to the posterior compartment of the thigh. Inferiorly, it divides to form the tibial nerve, continues into the popliteal fossa, and the common peroneal nerve, which passes laterally along the inferior border of the tendon of biceps femoris
- nerve to **obturator internus and superior gamellus**
- nerve to **quadratus femoris and inferior gamellus**
- **pudendal nerve** (S_2–S_4) passes over the ischial spine and back into the pelvis *via* the lesser sciatic notch (Fig. 3.37.1).

Back of thigh and popliteal fossa

The hamstrings, semitendinosus, semimembranosus and biceps femoris extend the hip and flex the knee. They are supplied by the sciatic nerve and perforating branches of the profunda femoris artery. They arise from the ischial tuberosity and attach distally to the tibia. Their tendons form the superior boundaries of the diamond-shaped **popliteal fossa** behind the knee (Figs 3.50.1–3.50.3). The medial and lateral heads of gastrocnemius form the inferior boundaries. Fascia lata is thickened to form the roof of the fossa, which supports and protects the neurovascular contents. The tibial nerve is most superficial, with the popliteal vein and popliteal artery lying close to the femur.

 INTRAMUSCULAR INJECTIONS IN THE BUTTOCK

As it emerges from the sciatic foramen, the sciatic nerve lies midway between the posterior superior iliac spine and the ischial tuberosity. As it leaves the gluteal region, the nerve lies midway between the ischial tuberosity and the greater trochanter. Intramuscular injections should always be given into the upper outer quadrant of the buttock in order to avoid the nerve.

47. Hip joint

Questions
- Why is the blood supply to the head of the femur important?
- What factors contribute to the stability of the hip?
- Why is the iliofemoral ligament one of the strongest ligaments of the body?

The hip joint is a synovial, ball and socket joint that allows a wide range of movement. It is very stable and is able to support the entire body weight during walking, running and jumping. When standing upright, the weight of the body falls behind the hip and so there is a tendency for the trunk to tip backwards at this joint (Fig. 3.41.2).

Powerful muscles lying anterior to the joint bring about flexion, adduction and medial rotation of the femur. Posteriorly and laterally, the gluteal and hamstring muscles act to cause extension, abduction and lateral rotation.

Stability
Stability of the hip is largely a consequence of the shape of the articular surfaces (Figs 3.47.1 and 3.47.2); traumatic injury, therefore, is likely to result in a fracture rather than damage to ligaments. Factors that ensure its stability—bony, ligamentous and muscular— also restrict its range of movement.

Bony features
The head of the femur is two-thirds of a sphere and is almost entirely enclosed by the acetabulum and its fibrocartilagenous labrum (Fig. 3.47.2). The femoral head and the lunate articular surface of the acetabulum are covered by hyaline cartilage. Osteoarthritis causes thinning of this cartilage and is visible on radiographs as reduction of the 'joint space'. The head faces upwards medially and forwards. The neck is approximately 5 cm long and set at an angle of 125° to the shaft (less in females). The narrowness of the femoral neck increases the range of possible movements but it also increases the stresses in that region, and fractures of the neck are fairly common particularly in the elderly.

Ligamentous features
The synovial capsule is tight and strong (Figs 3.47.3 and 3.47.4). Proximally, it is attached around the margins of the acetabulum and is lined by synovial membrane. Distally, the capsule attaches to the intertrochanteric line of the femur on its anterior surface and posteriorly it is attached to the neck of the femur about 1 cm short of the trochanteric crest (Fig. 3.37.1). Here the capsular (or retinacular) fibres turn back onto the neck, binding retinacular blood vessels tightly on the neck (Fig. 3.47.4).

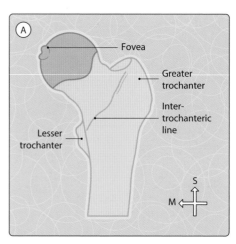

Fig. 3.47.1 The proximal part of the femur. (A) Anterior view; (B) posterior view.

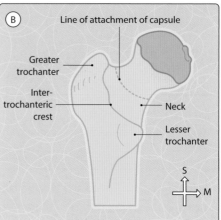

Fig. 3.47.2 Lateral view of acetabulum showing the labrum and transverse ligament.

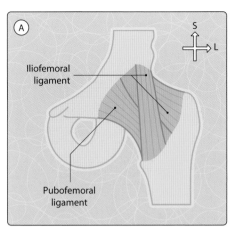

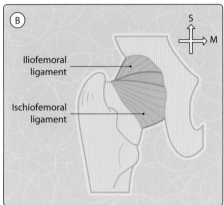

Fig. 3.47.3 The capsule of the hip joint. (A) Anterior view; (B) posterior view.

The capsule is thickened to form three intrinsic ligaments that are some of the strongest ligaments in the body (Fig. 3.47.3). The **iliofemoral ligament** strengthens the joint anteriorly, preventing hyperextension and supporting the body weight in the upright position. Posteriorly, the capsule is reinforced by the **pubofemoral** and **ischiofemoral ligaments**.

Muscular features

The joint is surrounded and supported on all aspects by powerful muscles.

Blood supply

The blood supply to the head of the femur comes from three sources:

- vessels within the shaft of the femur
- gluteal vessels and branches of the profunda femoris and obturator arteries contribute to the trochanteric and cruciate anastomoses, which supply the region of the hip joint and the head of the femur
- in children the femoral head also receives a supply from a branch of the obturator artery through the ligament of the head (ligamentum teres), which attaches to the fovea or pit of the femoral head (Fig. 3.47.4); this supply becomes less important after puberty.

Nerve supply

Branches of the obturator, femoral and sciatic nerves supply both the hip and knee joints. Pain caused by osteoarthritis of the hip may be referred to the knee. Patients complaining of knee pain should also have their hip examined.

 FRACTURE OF THE NECK OF FEMUR

The vessels supplying the head of the femur are bound tightly to the femoral neck by the retinacular fibres of the capsule. Fracture of the neck usually ruptures these vessels, resulting in avascular necrosis of the femoral head. In such cases, it is common to replace the femoral head with a metal prosthesis (hemiarthroplasty).

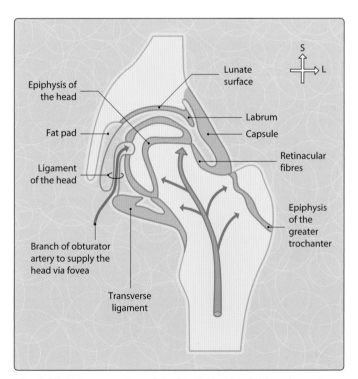

Fig. 3.47.4 Cross-section of the hip joint of a child to show the blood supply.

48. Knee joint

Questions
- In which position is the knee most stable? Can you explain why?
- What is the function of the posterior cruciate ligament?
- Which meniscus is most likely to be damaged?

The knee is a hinge joint that also allows some rotation. It is remarkably stable particularly in extension. The bony articulations between the condyles of the femur and tibia and the femur and patella provide no real stability (Fig. 3.48.1). It is supported primarily by its surrounding powerful muscles. Strong ligaments lie both within the capsule and outside and are important in supporting the knee in flexion and extension.

Capsule

The joint is enclosed posteriorly and laterally by the capsule and its synovial lining. Anteriorly, however, the capsule is deficient and is replaced by the quadriceps tendon, patella and patellar ligament. The synovial membrane passes under the quadriceps to become continuous with the **suprapatellar bursa** (Fig. 3.48.2). There are numerous other bursae around the knee, which may become inflamed and swollen. The capsule is perforated posterolateraly by the tendon of popliteus.

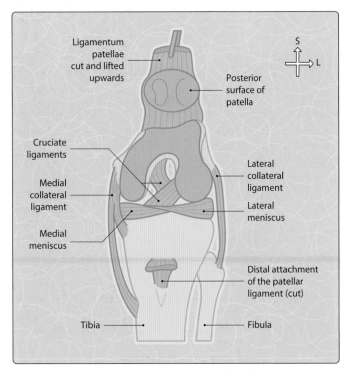

Fig. 3.48.1 Anterior view of the interior of the flexed knee joint with patella reflected superiorly.

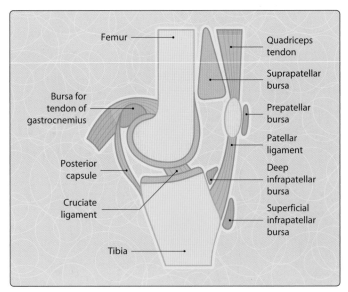

Fig. 3.48.2 Sagittal section of the knee showing the position of the bursae.

Ligaments

The ligaments play a major role in stabilizing the knee joint.

Intracapsular ligaments

The cruciate ligaments are extremely strong and join the femur to the tibia within the capsule. They cross each other like an X from both anterior and lateral aspects.

The **posterior cruciate ligament** is taut in flexion and supports the body weight when walking down a slope, i.e. it prevents the femur sliding forwards on the tibia (Figs 3.48.1, 3.48.3 and 3.48.4). It passes from a posterior tibial attachment to

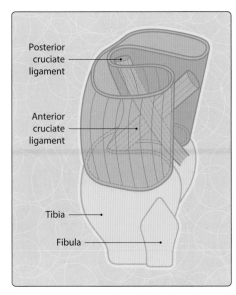

Fig. 3.48.3 Lateral oblique view of the knee joint showing the arrangement of the synovial membrane.

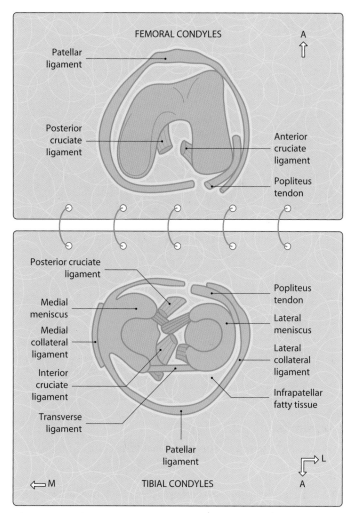

Fig. 3.48.4 The interior of the knee in the flexed position, with the capsule opened to show the attachments of the menisci.

its <u>a</u>nterior attachment to the intercondylar area of the femur and crosses <u>i</u>nternally: remember **PAIN.**

The **anterior cruciate ligament** is taut in extension and prevents the femur from sliding backwards on the tibia (Figs 3.48.1, 3.48.3 and 3.48.4). It passes from an <u>a</u>nterior tibial attachment to its <u>p</u>osterior attachment to the intercondylar area of the femur and crosses <u>ex</u>ternally: remember **APEX.**

Extracapsular ligaments

The **patellar ligament** is the continuation of the tendon of quadriceps below the patella (Figs 3.48.1 and 3.48.4).

The **lateral (fibular) collateral ligament** is a cord-like band attached from the lateral femoral condyle to the head of the fibula. It has no attachment to the lateral meniscus or the capsule (the tendon of popliteus lies deep to it). It is taut in extension and prevents adduction of the knee.

The **medial (tibial) collateral ligament** is a strong flat band thickening the capsule between the medial epicondyle of the femur and the tibia. It is attached to the medial meniscus, is taut in extension and prevents abduction.

The **oblique popliteal ligament** is an expansion of the tendon of semimembranosus that strengthens the back of the capsule (Fig. 3.50.2, p. 000).

Menisci

The **medial** and **lateral menisci** (semilunar, C-shaped fibrocartilages) act as cushions between the tibia and femur (Figs 3.48.1 and 3.48.4). They are attached to the capsule and by their ends to the intercondylar area of the **tibia**. The menisci are only torn when the knee is flexed and can rotate, such as when a footballer twists his flexed knee. Damage to the cartilage causes 'locking' of the knee because it is trapped between the articular surfaces. The medial meniscus is more commonly injured in twisting injuries, because its movement is restricted by its attachment to the medial collateral ligament.

Blood supply

The knee is supplied by an anastomosis formed by the genicular branches of the popliteal artery, obturator and femoral arteries (p. 110).

Nerve supply

The knee is supplied by the femoral, obturator and tibial nerves (p. 113). Patients may present with knee pain that is referred from the hip.

Movements

Extension involves the quadriceps (L_3, L_4); **flexion** involves the hamstrings (sciatic nerve L_5, S_1) and **rotation** occurs passively at the end of extension. The medial condyle of the femur is longer than the lateral and this allows a greater range of extension (think of the medial condyle as having 'tread'). This causes medial rotation of the femur on the tibia and *tightens all the major ligaments*. This 'locking' of the joint gives stability in extension without muscular activity. By comparison, unlocking the joint before flexion requires active contraction of popliteus to bring about lateral rotation of the femur.

 KNEE INJURIES

The knee is commonly injured because it is a major weight-bearing joint and its stability is dependent upon ligaments and muscles. With the foot weight bearing and, therefore, fixed on the ground, a hard blow to the *lateral* side of the knee causes:
- rupture of medial collateral ligament, opening the joint on the medial side
- tearing of the medial meniscus (because it is firmly attached to the medial collateral ligament)
- rupture of the anterior cruciate ligament.
Think of the 3Cs: <u>c</u>ollateral ligaments, <u>c</u>artilages and <u>c</u>ruciates

49. Anterior leg and dorsum of foot

Questions
- In which compartment are the muscles that extend the toes?
- In which compartment are the dorsiflexors of the ankle joint?
- Which bones articulate at the ankle joint?

The leg (Fig. 3.49.1) is surrounded by a dense stocking of fascia lata. A tough **interosseous membrane** between the tibia and fibula and a **posterior intermuscular septum** divide the leg into anterior and posterior compartments. The anterior compartment is further subdivided into anterior and lateral compartments by the **anterior intermuscular septum** (Fig. 3.49.2).

The compartments in the leg are particularly important. Because of the dense, inelastic fascia lata surrounding the calf muscles, muscle contraction in the posterior compartment squeezes the venous plexus within soleus. The presence of valves in the deep veins ensures that the movement of blood is

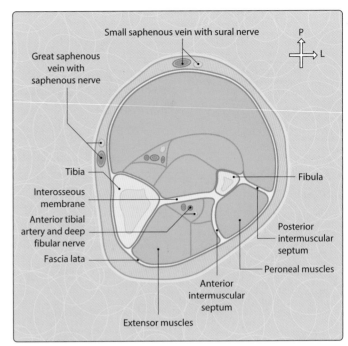

Fig. 3.49.2 Cross-section of the leg to show the anterior and lateral compartments.

upwards against the force of gravity. This mechanism aids venous return to the trunk and is known as the **calf muscle pump**. Compartment syndrome may result from a traumatic injury that causes haemorrhage into the confined space of the compartment (see p. 108).

The posterior compartment contains muscles that plantarflex the ankle joint and flex the toes; they are supplied by the tibial nerve. The anterior compartment contains muscles that dorsiflex the ankle, invert the foot at the subtalar joint and extend the toes; they are supplied by the deep branch of the common fibular nerve. The lateral compartment contains muscles that plantarflex the ankle and evert the foot; they are supplied by the superficial branch of the common fibular nerve.

Anterior (extensor) compartment
Remember that the leg is medially rotated compared with the upper limb, bringing the big toe to the medial position. The tendons of the four *extensor* muscles pass across the dorsum of the foot. This is equivalent to the extensor muscles of the *forearm* crossing the dorsum of the hand (notice that thin skin and a dorsal venous arch are characteristic of both the dorsum of the foot and the dorsum of the hand).

Where they pass beneath the extensor retinacula (Fig. 3.49.1), the tendons are enclosed in synovial sheaths.

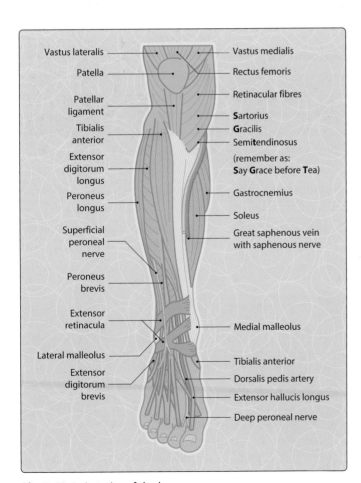

Fig. 3.49.1 Anterior of the leg.

The muscles are:

- **tibialis anterior**: most medial; it dorsiflexes the ankle and inverts the foot at the subtalar joint
- **extensor hallucis longus**: dorsiflexes and extends the big toe
- **extensor digitorum longus**: dorsiflexes and extends the lateral four toes
- **peroneus tertius**: functionally unimportant.

Extension of the digits is assisted by a small muscle on the dorsum of the foot, the **extensor digitorum brevis** (Fig. 3.49.1).

Arterial and nerve supply

The anterior and lateral compartments are supplied by the **common fibular nerve** (L_4, L_5, S_1, S_2), one of the terminal branches of the sciatic nerve. In the popliteal fossa, it lies along the inferior border of the tendon of biceps femoris and passes laterally around the neck of the fibula, pierces peroneus longus and divides into superficial and deep branches.

The muscles are supplied by the **deep branch of the fibular nerve** (L_4, L_5, S_1). It terminates by supplying a small area of skin in the cleft between the first and second toes. The compartment is supplied by the **anterior tibial artery**, which is a terminal branch of the popliteal artery. It continues distal to the ankle as the dorsalis pedis artery. The pulse of the dorsalis pedis artery can be felt lateral to the tendon of extensor hallucis longus.

Lateral (fibular) compartment

Two muscles pass posterior to the lateral malleolus where they are held in place by the peroneal retinacula (Fig. 3.49.3). Their actions are plantiflexion and eversion (abduction) of the subtalar joint.

Peroneus longus is superficial; its tendon crosses under the foot in a bony groove to attach to the base of the first metatarsal. It supports the lateral arch of the foot (p. 126).

Peroneus brevis is attached to the base of the fifth metatarsal.

Arterial and nerve supply

The lateral compartment supplied by the **superficial fibular nerve** (L_4, L_5, S_1), which terminates by supplying the skin of the front of the leg and the dorsum of the foot. It is also supplied by the fibular branch of the tibial artery.

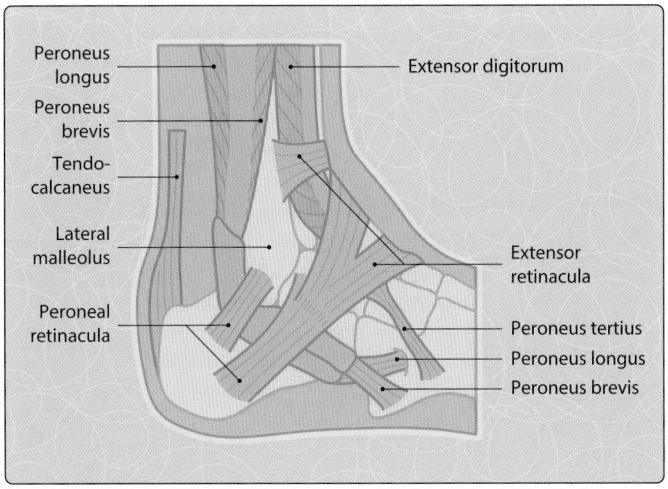

Peroneus longus
Peroneus brevis
Tendocalcaneus
Lateral malleolus
Peroneal retinacula
Extensor digitorum
Extensor retinacula
Peroneus tertius
Peroneus longus
Peroneus brevis

Fig. 3.49.3 Lateral view of the ankle region to show the tendons of the peroneal muscles.

 DAMAGE TO THE COMMON PERONEAL NERVE

In the upper limb, there are three important nerves that lie in direct contact with the humerus and are vulnerable to damage if the bone is fractured (p. 44). In the lower limb, the only nerve that is vulnerable in this way is the common fibular nerve as it winds around the lateral aspect of the neck of the fibula. Damage results in loss of innervation to the lateral (peroneal) and anterior (extensor) compartments, affecting dorsiflexion, eversion and toe extension and leading to the development of a condition known as foot drop.

50. Posterior leg

Questions
- Which muscles in the leg are important for normal venous return from the lower limb?
- Which structures pass posterior to the medial malleolus?

Posterior (flexor) compartment

There are two layers of muscles in the posterior (flexor) compartment of the leg; they have very important functions in gait and posture as well as being essential for normal venous return from the lower limbs (Figs 3.50.1 and 3.50.2).

Remember the sole of the foot is equivalent to the palm of the hand; both are covered in thick skin that protects arterial arches and nerves. This tip will help you to recall that the long *flexors* of the toes lie in the calf, pass behind the ankle and cross the sole of the foot, just like the long flexors of the fingers lie in the palm.

Superficial layer

The three muscles of the superficial layer (Fig. 3.50.1) are plantiflexors of the ankle and have a common powerful tendon (tendocalcaneus or **Achilles tendon**) that attaches to the calcaneus.

Gastrocnemius has two heads that arise from the epicondyles of the femur. It flexes the knee and is a powerful plantiflexor of the ankle.

Soleus is a powerful muscle important in normal walking and running ('stroll with soleus'). There is a deep venous plexus within soleus. The soleus muscle stabilizes the tibia on the calcaneus, limiting forward sway (Fig. 3.50.3).

Plantaris lies between the other two muscles. It is small and may be absent.

The line of gravity falling in front of the ankle creates a tendency to sway forward at the ankle (Fig. 3.41.2). When you are standing, soleus and gastrocnemius contract regularly, which plantiflexes the ankle and counteracts the effects of gravity, maintaining an upright posture (Fig. 3.50.1A). Contractions of gastrocnemius and soleus assist the return of venous blood from the lower limbs (**calf muscle pump**, p. 122).

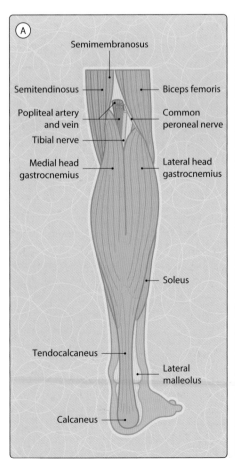
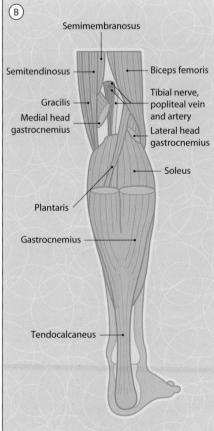
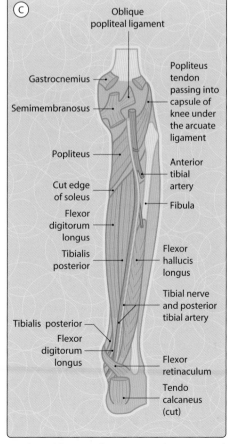

Fig. 3.50.1 Posterior view of the muscles of the calf. (A) Superficial muscles; (B) Superficial muscles with part of gastrocnemius removed; (C) deep muscles with superficial muscles removed.

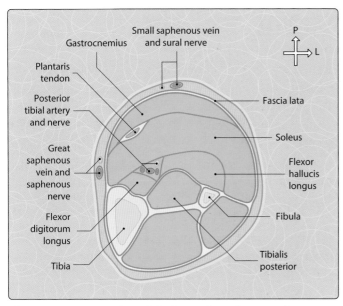

Fig. 3.50.2 Cross-section of the leg to show the posterior compartments.

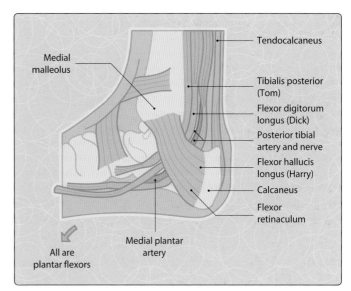

Fig. 3.50.3 Plantar flexion by soleus muscle limits forward sway.

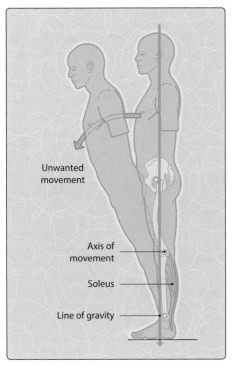

Fig. 3.50.4 Medial view of the ankle region to show the tendons of the deep calf muscles.

(The order of tendons of these muscles passing behind the medial malleolus can be remembered as <u>T</u>om, <u>D</u>ick and <u>H</u>arry.) The tendons of these muscles are held in position by the flexor retinaculum (Fig. 3.50.4) and enclosed in synovial sheaths that sometimes become inflamed in athletes.

Arterial and nerve supply

The neurovascular bundle containing the tibial nerve and posterior tibial artery lies between the deep and superficial groups of muscles.

All the muscles of the posterior compartment are supplied by the **tibial nerve** (L_4, L_5, S_1–S_3). It also gives articular branches and the **sural nerve,** which accompanies the small saphenous vein and supplies the skin on the lateral side of the calf and foot. The tibial nerve passes behind the medial malleolus (Fig. 3.50.4) and divides to give its terminal branches, the **medial** and **lateral plantar nerves,** which supply the muscles of the foot. The **posterior tibial artery** is the continuation of the popliteal artery; it gives a peroneal branch and its pulse can be felt between the medial malleolus and the calcaneus.

Deep layer

There are four muscles in the deep layer:

■ **popliteus** acts on the knee joint (p. 121)
■ **tibialis posterior** lies deepest, passes behind the medial malleolus; it plantiflexes and inverts the foot
■ **flexor digitorum longus** has four tendons that insert into the phalanges of the lateral four toes
■ **flexor hallucis longus** is a more powerful muscle that inserts into the terminal phalanx of the big toe; it is vital in the final push-off for running.

RUPTURE OF THE ACHILLES TENDON

If the Achilles tendon is ruptured, running is impossible and walking severely affected because the gastrocnemius and soleus muscles plantiflex the ankle, raising the weight of the body up onto the toes for the 'push-off' phase of walking and running. Tapping the Achilles tendon tests the tibial nerve and spinal segments S_1 and S_2.

51. Bones of the foot and ankle joint

Questions
- What are the possible movements at the ankle joint?
- Which bones articulate at the subtalar joint?
- What structures support the medial longitudinal arch?

The foot supports the entire body weight and provides an elastic but stable platform for movement. A series of bony arches spread the body weight and act as shock absorbers.

Arches of the foot

A footprint shows exactly how the foot supports the body weight: the heel, lateral border of the foot, heads of the metatarsals (especially the first) and the tips of the toes.

Body weight transfers from the tibia and talus to the calcaneus posteriorly and to navicular, cuneiforms and metatarsals anteriorly. These bones make up the **longitudinal arch**, which is subdivided into medial and lateral parts (Fig. 3.51.1). The **medial longitudinal arch** is higher and is maintained by the pull of tibialis anterior from above. The tarsal bones lock into position under stress with the talus as the keystone of the arch supported inferiorly by the spring ligament. The plantar aponeurosis acts as a tie beam between the proximal and distal ends of the arch

(Fig. 3.52.1, p. 128) and its tension changes in different positions of the foot. The **lateral arch** rests on the ground during standing (Fig. 3.51.2).

The **transverse arch** is maintained by the wedge-shaped cuneiforms and the bases of the metatarsals. They are tightly bound together by ligaments and the tendon of peroneus longus as it crosses the sole of the foot from lateral to medial (Fig. 3.52.1).

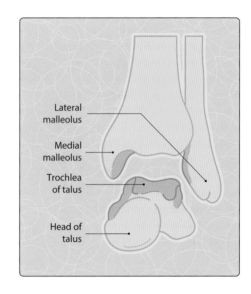

Fig. 3.51.2 Anterior view of the bones of the ankle joint.

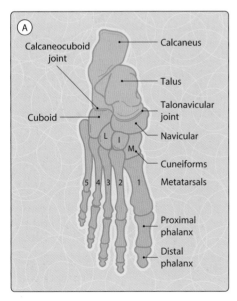

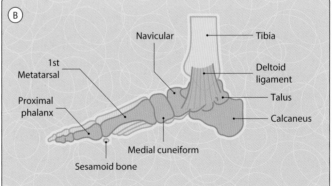

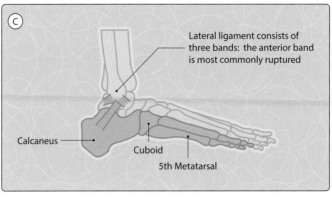

Fig. 3.51.1 Bones of the foot. (A) From above; (B) medial view to show the medial longitudinal arch (in blue); (C) lateral view to show the lateral ligaments and longitudinal arch (in blue).

Ankle joint

The ankle joint is a simple hinge that allows only **plantiflexion** and **dorsiflexion.** The distal ends of the tibia and fibula are united by a strong interosseous ligament that creates a mortise into which the talus fits, forming the ankle joint (Fig. 3.51.2). The talus is wider anteriorly and becomes firmly wedged between the malleoli in dorsiflexion (thus the ankle is least stable when plantiflexed). The capsule and the medial (deltoid) and lateral collateral ligaments of the ankle are strong but are frequently sprained, particularly on the lateral side (Fig. 3.51.1b,c). Fractures around the ankle are common, but the joint rarely dislocates.

Other joints

There are a number of other joints in the foot between tarsals, metatarsals and phalanges. Walking involves a series of events requiring all these joints (Fig. 3.51.3). Walking on uneven ground involves rotational movements of the foot:

- **eversion** by muscles of the lateral compartment of the leg, peroneus longus and brevis (superficial peroneal nerve)
- **inversion** by muscles attached to the medial side of the foot, tibialis anterior, tibialis posterior, extensor hallucis longus (tibial nerve).

The following joints allow eversion and inversion:

- **subtalar** or **talocalcanear joint** (Fig. 3.51.4): a gliding joint underneath the body of the talus and the upper surface of the calcaneus
- **talocalcaneonavicular joint**: a complex ball and socket joint between the head of the talus and a socket formed by the posterior aspect of the navicular and the sustentaculum tali of the calcaneus; the navicular and calcaneus are tied together by the plantar calcaneonavicular or **spring ligament**
- **calcaneocuboid joint**: a separate joint but functions with the talocalcaneonavicular joint (sometimes called the mid-tarsal joint).

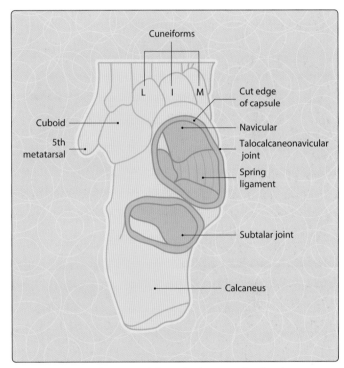

Fig. 3.51.4 Attachments of the articular capsules for the talocalcanear and talocalcaneonavicular joints; viewed from above with the talus removed.

Fig. 3.51.3
Sequence of events between heel strike and push off.
1, Heel strike, the ankle plantar flexes;
2, weight rolls along the lateral border;
3, the metatarso-phalangeal joints flex to give 'push off'; 4, final push off is from big toe and flexor hallucis longus; 5, foot leaves the ground, the ankle dorsiflexes to clear toes and the hip swings forward.

SPRAINED ANKLE AND POTT'S FRACTURE

The ankle is the most frequently injured major joint. A sprained ankle results from twisting the weight-bearing foot and is usually an inversion injury. Fibres of the lateral ligament may be torn.

Forced eversion damages the very strong deltoid ligament, which may tear off the medial malleolus; the talus dislocates laterally and fractures the fibula. This is known as a Pott's fracture.

52. Sole of the foot

Question
- Why is it difficult to give a local anaesthetic in the sole of the foot?

You do not need a detailed knowledge of the anatomy of the foot; it is less often damaged than the hand. Remember that the organization of the sole of the foot is very similar to the palm of the hand.

The sole is covered in **thick skin** tightly attached to deep tissues. The **superficial fascia** consists of dense fatty tissue forming cushions over weight-bearing areas. Fibrous septa divide it into pockets, which make it difficult to infiltrate local anaesthetic and in which infections may develop.

The **plantar aponeurosis** (sometimes plantar fascia) (Fig. 3.52.1) is a thickened layer of deep fascia equivalent to the palmar aponeurosis. It acts as a tie bar for the longitudinal arch attached between the calcaneus and the proximal phalanges (Fig. 3.51.1). It becomes rigid when you 'push off' with your foot, pulling the ends of the longitudinal arch together. Pull your toes up (extension) and you can see and feel the aponeurosis tighten along the sole of your foot.

The muscles are equivalent to those in the hand; they help to maintain the arches of the foot, but it is not necessary to most people to have individual control of their toes.

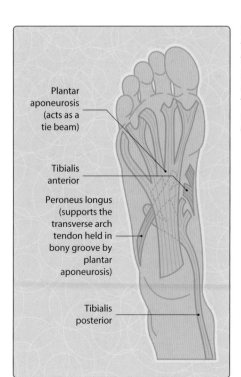

Plantar aponeurosis (acts as a tie beam)

Tibialis anterior

Peroneus longus (supports the transverse arch tendon held in bony groove by plantar aponeurosis)

Tibialis posterior

Fig. 3.52.1 Sole of foot showing the tendons of peroneus longus and tibialis anterior forming a stirrup to support the arches of the foot.

Layers
Other structures of the sole of foot are described in layers (Fig. 3.52.2).

First layer
The first layer of the foot consists of **flexor digitorum brevis** (equivalent to flexor digitorum superficialis of the hand) and **abductors** of the big and little toes.

Second layer
The second layer consists of neurovascular structures. The tibial nerve (L_4, L_5, S_1, S_2) and posterior tibial artery pass behind the medial malleolus and divide to give their terminal branches.

The **medial plantar nerve** (L_4, L_5) and its branches are accompanied by the **medial plantar artery**. The medial plantar nerve is equivalent to the *median* nerve in the hand. It gives motor branches to the short muscles of the big toe and the medial lumbrical and cutaneous branches to the medial 3½ toes. It also supplies the flexor digitorum brevis.

The **lateral plantar nerve** (S_1, S_2) passes with the **lateral plantar artery** to the base of the little toe and, like the ulnar nerve in the hand, gives a deep motor branch to all the other short muscles of the foot and a superficial cutaneous branch to the lateral 1½ toes. The lateral plantar artery passes deeply and forms the deep plantar arch, which anastomoses with a branch of the dorsalis pedis artery.

Third layer
The third layer is made up of the **long flexor tendons** with **lumbricals** and **flexor accessories**.

Fourth layer
The fourth layer contains the **flexor hallucis brevis.** It has two bellies with a sesamoid bone in each tendon. They articulate directly with the base of the first metatarsal. The sesamoid bones form a channel for the tendon of flexor hallucis longus. This layer also has **adductor hallucis** and the **short flexor of the little toe**.

Fifth layer
The fifth layer contains the deep branches of lateral plantar nerve and the plantar arch.

Sixth layer
The sixth layer comprises the **interossei**, the tendons of **peroneus longus** and **tibialis posterior** and important ligaments of the foot, including the long and short plantar ligaments and the deep transverse metacarpal ligament, which helps to support the transverse arch.

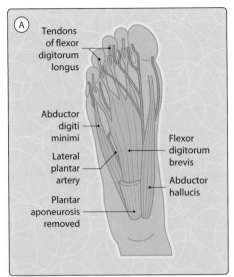

A
Tendons of flexor digitorum longus
Abductor digiti minimi
Lateral plantar artery
Plantar aponeurosis removed
Flexor digitorum brevis
Abductor hallucis

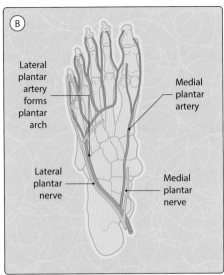

B
Lateral plantar artery forms plantar arch
Lateral plantar nerve
Medial plantar artery
Medial plantar nerve

Fig. 3.52.2 Sole of the right foot. (A) The first layer; (B) the second layer showing the neurovascular supply; (C) the third layer, showing the long flexors and lumbrical muscles; (D) the fourth layer; (E) the sixth layer of the right foot.

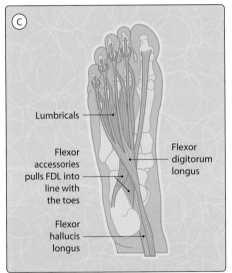

C
Lumbricals
Flexor accessories pulls FDL into line with the toes
Flexor hallucis longus
Flexor digitorum longus

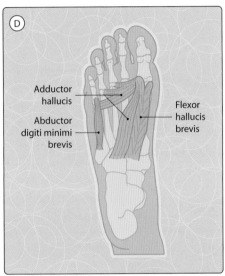

D
Adductor hallucis
Abductor digiti minimi brevis
Flexor hallucis brevis

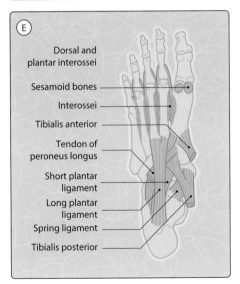

E
Dorsal and plantar interossei
Sesamoid bones
Interossei
Tibialis anterior
Tendon of peroneus longus
Short plantar ligament
Long plantar ligament
Spring ligament
Tibialis posterior

BLEEDING FROM THE FOOT

Bleeding from the plantar arch may be severe. It is difficult to control because the arch lies deep to the dense plantar aponeurosis and flexor digitorum brevis.

53. Review of the nerve supply and clinical testing

Questions
- What nerve problems give rise to clinical signs in the lower limb?
- How do you test for nerve damage?

Problems related to the nerve roots of L_1–S_4 will give rise to clinical signs in the lower limb (Table 3.53.1). Clinical testing of these nerve roots involves the examination of the myotomes, tendon reflexes of the limb and the dermatomes.

Motor distribution
Myotomes can be tested if spinal (central) damage is suspected:

L_3, L_4: hip flexion adduction medial rotation

L_5, S_1: hip extension, abduction lateral rotation

L_3, L_4: knee extension (knee jerk reflex)

L_5, S_1: knee flexion

L_4, L_5: ankle dorsiflexion

S_1, S_2: ankle plantiflexion (ankle jerk reflex)

L_4: foot inversion

L_5, S_1: foot eversion.

Spinal segments can be tested:

L_1, L_2: skin front of thigh

L_3, L_4: knee jerk, skin over patella

L_5: skin lateral side of leg and foot

S_1, S_2: ankle jerk, skin lateral side of foot and back of thigh

S_3, S_4: skin over buttocks and perianal region.

Sensory distribution
During development, the lower limb rotates medially bringing the big toe into the midline. This is the reason why the dermatomes spiral around the limb. Dermatomes are tested when spinal (central) damage is suspected. The dermatomes and test areas are:

L_3: anterior surface of knee (3 the knee)

S_2: popliteal fossa

L_5: under the big toe (remember 5 under 1)

S_1: under the little toe (remember 1 under 5).

Peripheral nerves arising from the lumbosacral plexus are tested by their cutaneous distribution:

femoral: skin over anterior thigh, knee jerk

obturator: skin over medial thigh, hip adduction

tibial: ankle jerk

deep peroneal: dorsiflexion

superficial peroneal: skin over dorsum foot and eversion.

Table 3.53.1 SITES OF POSSIBLE NERVE DAMAGE

Site of damage	Nerve	Motor effect	Sensory loss
Anterior superior iliac spine	Compression of the lateral cutaneous nerve of thigh		Paraesthesia over the lateral thigh, known as meralgia paraesthetica
Posterior dislocation of hip	Sciatic nerve	Paralysis of the hamstrings and all the muscles of leg and foot	Lateral side of foot and leg
Misplaced intramuscular injection in gluteal region	Sciatic nerve	Paralysis of the hamstrings and all the muscles of leg and foot	Lateral side of foot and leg
Popliteal fossa	Tibial and/or common peroneal nerve	Paralysis of all the muscles of the leg and foot	Lateral side of foot and leg
Neck of fibula; compression by a tight plaster cast	Common peroneal nerve	'Foot drop' (loss of eversion and dorsiflexion)	Loss of sensation over dorsum of foot
Procedures involving the great saphenous vein can damage saphenous nerve			Loss of sensation over the medial leg and foot

DIABETIC NEUROPATHY: THE DIABETIC FOOT

Diabetes is a common disease that is caused by insulin deficiency. It affects 120 million people worldwide and has serious effects on health partly through damage to the cardiovascular and nervous systems.

It affects large vessels causing coronary artery disease, stroke and peripheral vascular disease. Damage to small vessels results in very serious damage to the kidneys, retina and peripheral nerves.

Hyperglycaemia caused by diabetes damages peripheral nervous tissue in a number of ways. The earliest changes affect the myelin sheaths, which leads to degeneration of the nerve axons (neuropathy). Several forms of neuropathy are associated with diabetes. However, the *general* effects neatly illustrate the function of mixed peripheral nerves that consist of motor, sensory and sympathetic fibres. Damage to nerves leads to anaesthesia, paralysis and atrophy.

Sensory damage

Damage to cutaneous nerves results in **anaesthesia** over the foot and lower leg involving what is sometimes described as the 'stocking area' (loss of sensation in the hands is less common). Numbness of the feet means that patients may be unaware that they have burnt themselves on a hot-water bottle or that ill-fitting shoes are causing blisters. Other sensory functions that will be affected include loss of vibration sense, pain and proprioception in the joints of the feet. Without this positional information from the foot, it becomes difficult to balance and walking damages the joints of the feet with resulting pain and deformity (Charcot's joints).

Motor damage

Loss of motor control of the small muscles of the feet leads to **paralysis** and muscle wasting (**atrophy**) and clawing of the toes. The muscles of the leg may also become involved and changes in gait lead to callus formation under the foot that eventually ulcerates.

Sympathetic damage

The skin receives sympathetic neurones that constrict superficial blood vessels and cause sweating. An area of skin affected by a peripheral neuropathy will look pink and feel warm and dry since blood vessels will be dilated and sweating will be inhibited.

The diabetic foot

Foot problems are common in diabetic patients and result in frequent hospital admissions in this group. Diabetic ulcers commonly become infected through poor blood supply and glucose-saturated tissues. Vascular insufficiency plus infection lead to gangrene and osteomyelitis, necessitating amputation.

54. The skull

Questions
- Why are the bones of the face and cranium so different?
- What major structure passes through the foramen magnum?
- Which bones contain air sinuses?

The skull consists of the cranium and facial skeleton (Figs 3.54.1–3.54.3). It is a complex three-dimensional arrangement of 21 bones that meet at fixed fibrous joints known as **sutures**. The only synovial joint is the **temporomandibular joint** (TM joint) where the head of the mandible articulates with the temporal bone (Fig. 3.54.2).

Cranium

The **cranium** or vault of the skull protects the brain. It is made up of flat bones consisting of spongy bone containing red bone marrow (**diploë**) sandwiched between two plates of compact bone. The cranium is strongest posteriorly (**occiput**) and weakest at the **pterion** over the temple (Fig. 3.54.2).

The cranium is formed by four pairs of bones.

1. **Frontal bones** normally fuse to form the forehead and the superior margins of the orbits. The frontal sinuses lie in the roof of the orbit (Fig. 3.64.2).
2. **Parietal bones** meet in the midline of the sagittal suture. Anteriorly, they meet the sphenoid at the pterion and

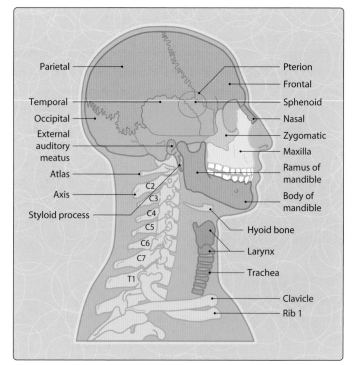

Fig. 3.54.2 Lateral view of the bones of the skull and the cervical spine.

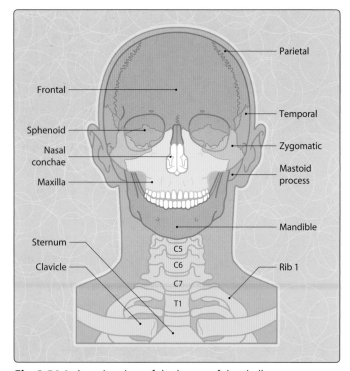

Fig. 3.54.1 Anterior view of the bones of the skull.

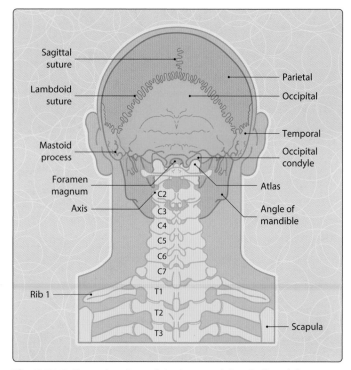

Fig. 3.54.3 Posterior view of the bones of the skull and the cervical spine.

posteriorly form the lambdoid suture with the occipital bones. Internally, the parietal bones are marked by the meningeal vessels. The markings may be visible in radiographs and could be mistaken for a fracture line (Fig. 3.57.1).

3. **Temporal bones** are described in five parts:
   - **squamous,** with the external auditory foramen
   - **tympanic plate** and mandibular fossa (articular surface for the temporomandibular joint, p. 144)
   - **mastoid process,** which contains air cells directly connected to the middle ear
   - **petrous,** with the internal auditory meatus housing the organs of hearing and balance
   - **zygomatic process,** which forms a buttress with the zygoma of the facial skeleton.

4. **Occipital** is the thickest bone of the skull and forms the boundaries of the foramen magnum through which the spinal cord travels; nodding movements occur between the occipital condyles and the atlas (p. 28).

The face

The bones of the face are light and easily damaged; those forming the medial walls of the orbit are paper thin (p. 146). Fractures may damage the nerves or vessels that pass through bony canals (foramina) in the skull. The maxilla, frontal and ethmoid bones are hollow; they enclose the **paranasal air sinuses**: air spaces lined by respiratory epithelium that drain into the nasal cavity (p. 152). The most important facial bones are:

- **maxilla**: forms part of the middle part of the face; it is hollow (maxillary air sinus) and is very fragile; its alveolar process carries the teeth of the upper jaw and it also has the infraorbital foramen (Fig. 3.54.1)
- **sphenoid**: is a complex shape, forming the middle cranial fossa (p. 134), pituitary fossa, back of the orbit, pterion and lateral and medial pterygoid plates; the sphenoid encloses important foramina, the optic canal, superior and inferior orbital fissures, and the foramina rotundum, ovale and spinosum
- **ethmoid**: honeycomb of air sinuses that form the medial walls of the nasal cavity and orbit (Fig. 3.64.3, p. 153)
- **nasal**: forms the bridge of the nose
- **mandible**: major features are the body and mental foramen, ramus and mandibular foramen, angle, coronoid process, head (condyle) and neck (Fig. 3.64.2, p. 153).

NEONATAL SKULL AT BIRTH

A baby has a very large cranium relative to the size of its face because the maxillary air sinuses are tiny and the teeth have not yet erupted (Fig. 3.54.4). At birth, the bones of the cranium are not fully grown and are connected by fibrous membranes forming the **anterior** and **posterior fontanelles** (soft spots), which allow some compression of the skull during birth and for postnatal growth of the brain. They close during the first 2 years of life. The anterior fontanelle becomes depressed in a dehydrated baby and may bulge if there is raised intracranial pressure.

Because the mastoid process and tympanic plate of the temporal bone develop after birth, the facial nerve and eardrum (tympanic membrane) are more superficial and vulnerable to damage in neonates (take care with the otoscope when examining a baby for middle ear infections).

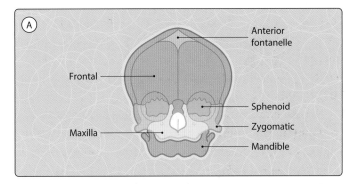

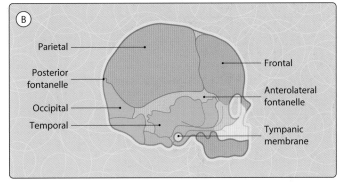

Fig. 3.54.4 The neonatal skull. (A) Anterior view; (B) lateral view.

55. Internal features of the cranium and the meninges

Questions
- Which lobes of the brain occupy the three cranial fossae?
- What structures lie in the subarachnoid space?
- What is the function of the arachnoid granulations?

The cranium

The cranium is marked internally by ridges for attachment of the **dura mater** (see below) and by meningeal vessels that supply the meninges and diploë. The cranial nerves and blood vessels that supply the brain pass through foramina in the skull (Table 3.55.1). There are also a variable number of foramina for the passage of **emissary veins** (Fig. 3.55.1), which connect intracranial and extracranial veins (they may allow infection to spread into the cranium).

The base of the skull supports the brain and is divided into three (Fig. 3.55.2).

1. The **anterior cranial fossa** is related to the frontal lobes of the brain and the olfactory bulbs. The floor is formed by the orbital plate of the frontal bone, lesser wing of sphenoid and the cribriform plate of the ethmoid. A fold of dura, the falx cerebri, is attached anteriorly to the crista galli.
2. The **middle cranial fossa** is occupied by the temporal lobes of the brain, part of the forebrain, the optic chiasma and the termination of the internal carotid arteries. The floor consists of the sphenoid, in which there are several important foramina, and the anterior part of the petrous temporal bone. In the midline, the body of the sphenoid forms the pituitary fossa where the pituitary lies.
3. The **posterior cranial fossa** is separated from the middle fossa by the petrous temporal bone; the floor is formed by the occipital bone and a dense layer of dura (tentorium cerebelli) forms a roof over it. The fossa houses the cerebellum, pons and medulla.

The meninges

The brain and spinal cord are enclosed by three membranes, the meninges. The major foramina and the structures that pass through them are listed in Table 3.55.1.

1. **Pia mater** is a delicate vascular membrane that closely follows all the complex folds on the surface of the brain.
2. **Arachnoid mater** is closely associated with the pia mater but does not dip down into the deep folds on the surface of the brain, leaving gaps between the pia and arachnoid. The larger arteries and veins of the brain lie in these **subarachnoid spaces** supported by **cerebrospinal fluid** (CSF) and a cobweb of fine filaments. CSF is secreted by the ependymal lining of the ventricles of the brain (choroid plexus); it fills the ventricles, the central canal of the spinal cord and the subarachnoid space surrounding the brain and spinal cord.

Table 3.55.1 THE CRANIAL FOSSAE AND FORAMINA

Cranial fossae	Foramen	Major contents	Communicates with
Anterior	Cribriform plate	Olfactory nerve (CN I)	Nasal cavity
Middle	Optic canal	Optic nerve (CN II) with meninges, ophthalmic artery	Orbit
	Superior orbital fissure	Oculomotor (CN III)	Orbit
		Trochlear (CN IV)	
		Trigeminal (ophthalmic; CN V$_a$)	
		Abducens, ophthalmic veins (CN VI)	
	Foramen rotundum	Trigeminal (maxillary; CN V$_b$)	Pterygopalatine fossa
	Foramen ovale	Trigeminal (mandibular; CN V$_c$); trigeminal motor root; emissary vein from cavernous sinus	Infratemporal fossa
	Foramen spinosum	Middle meningeal artery	
	Foramen lacerum filled with cartilage to form part of the carotid canal	Internal carotid artery carrying sympathetic plexus	
Posterior	Internal acoustic meatus	Facial (CN VII: motor root and nervus intermedius)	Stylomastoid foramen
		Vestibulocochlear (CN VIII)	Inner ear
	Jugular foramen	Glossopharyngeal (CN IX), vagus (CN X), accessory (CN XI); internal jugular vein	Neck
	Hypoglossal canal	Hypoglossal (CN XII)	Neck
	Foramen magnum	Medulla oblongata and meninges, vertebral and anterior and posterior spinal arteries, spinal part of CN X1	

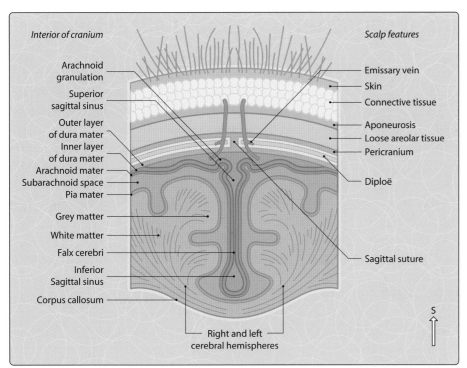

Interior of cranium   *Scalp features*

- Arachnoid granulation
- Superior sagittal sinus
- Outer layer of dura mater
- Inner layer of dura mater
- Arachnoid mater
- Subarachnoid space
- Pia mater
- Grey matter
- White matter
- Falx cerebri
- Inferior Sagittal sinus
- Corpus callosum

- Emissary vein
- Skin
- Connective tissue
- Aponeurosis
- Loose areolar tissue
- Pericranium
- Diploë
- Sagittal suture

S

Right and left cerebral hemispheres

Fig. 3.55.1 Coronal section of the scalp, skull and meninges showing the interior of the cranium and the scalp features. The scalp features can be remembered as SCALP: skin, connective tissue, aponeurosis, loose areolar tissue, pericranium.

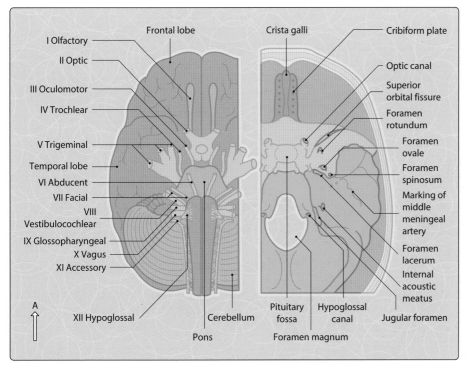

- I Olfactory
- II Optic
- III Oculomotor
- IV Trochlear
- V Trigeminal
- Temporal lobe
- VI Abducent
- VII Facial
- VIII Vestibulocochlear
- IX Glossopharyngeal
- X Vagus
- XI Accessory

- Frontal lobe
- Crista galli
- Cribiform plate
- Optic canal
- Superior orbital fissure
- Foramen rotundum
- Foramen ovale
- Foramen spinosum
- Marking of middle meningeal artery
- Foramen lacerum
- Internal acoustic meatus

A

- XII Hypoglossal
- Cerebellum
- Pons
- Pituitary fossa
- Foramen magnum
- Hypoglossal canal
- Jugular foramen

Fig. 3.55.2 Cranial nerve attachments to the base of the brain and the reciprocal skull base.

3. **Dura mater** is the tough membrane lining the inside of the cranium. There are two layers of dura; the outer layer is fused with the periosteum of the skull but in some specific areas, the inner and outer layers separate to enclose the **dural venous sinuses,** which drain blood from the brain (Figs 3.58.2 and 3.58.3). In the superior sagittal sinus (Fig. 3.55.1), there are defects in the dura that allow small protrusions of the arachnoid to billow into the sinus (**arachnoid granulations** or **villi**) allowing resorption of CSF into the venous system. They sometimes become calcified and can be identified in radiograph images as markers for the midline. The inner layer of dura is extended in some places to form folds that physically support the brain. The **falx cerebri** hangs down, partially separating the cerebral hemispheres. It attaches posteriorly to the **tentorium cerebelli,** which forms a shelf between the cerebellum and the posterior lobes of the cerebral hemispheres (p. 140).

Intracranial haemorrhages

There are several types of intracranial bleeds:

- **extradural**: a blow to the head can cause arterial bleeding between the skull and dura (e.g. at the pterion)
- **subdural**: a jolt to the head causes venous bleeding between the dura and arachnoid; this is most common in the elderly
- **subarachnoid**: bleeding into the CSF from arteries lying in the subarachnoid space (e.g. from the circle of Willis; p. 139); it is the commonest cause of death in young adults
- **cerebral**: bleeding from arteries within the substance of the brain (stroke).

56. Cranial nerves and sympathetic supply to the head

Questions
- Which cranial nerve supplies the muscles of facial expression?
- Which cranial nerves control the extraocular muscles?
- Which cranial nerves carry parasympathetic fibres?

The 12 cranial nerves are numbered in the order they arise from the brainstem. Table 3.56.1 details them and Figure 1.8 (p. 9) illustrates their roles. *You should know the important functions of these nerves and how to test them* (p. 160).

Sympathetic and parasympathetic supply to the head

Sympathetic neurones supplying the head or neck area arise in the lateral grey columns of spinal segments T1 and T2 (p. 74). Preganglionic fibres synapse in the superior cervical sympathetic ganglion and are carried on the surface of the internal carotid artery and its branches to the orbit and skin. Sympathetic stimulation brings about vasoconstriction of blood vessels, sweating and dilatation of the pupil. Levator palpebrae superiores is partially supplied by sympathetic nerves.

Parasympathetic neurones lie in the nuclei of four cranial nerves—III, VI, IX and X—and synapse in autonomic ganglia close to the organ being supplied (Table 3.56.1). The vagus is entirely parasympathetic and its neurones synapse in the organ supplied.

Table 3.56.1 THE 12 CRANIAL NERVES

Nerve	Origin, foramen and destination	Fibre types	Supply and function
I Olfactory	Nerve cells in the nasal cavity, roof, cribriform plate, olfactory bulb and tract to forebrain	Special sense	Nasal mucosa; smell
II Optic	Ganglion cells in retina form the optic nerve, optic canal, optic tract to forebrain	Special sense	Retina; vision
III Oculomotor	Ventral aspect of midbrain, lateral wall of cavernous sinus, superior orbital fissure Orbit	Motor	Extraocular muscles: levator palpebrae superioris, inferior oblique, superior, medial and inferior rectus and inferior obliques muscles
	Edinger–Westphal nucleus of the brainstem; travels with CN III to orbit; neurones synapse in ciliary ganglion	Parasympathetic	Smooth muscle of constrictor of the pupil (sphincter pupillae) and of ciliary body (focusing of the lens)
IV Trochlear	Dorsal aspect of midbrain, lateral wall of cavernous sinus, superior orbital fissure, orbit	Motor	Extraocular muscle, superior oblique
V Trigeminal: with three divisions	Pons of hindbrain, sensory ganglion in the trigeminal cave (middle cranial fossa)	Mixed	
Vₐ Ophthalmic	Lateral wall of cavernous sinus, superior orbital fissure, roof of the orbit	Sensory	Skin of scalp, forehead, upper eyelid and nose, cornea and conjunctiva (frontal, lacrimal and nasociliary branches)
V_b Maxillary	Lateral wall of cavernous sinus, foramen rotundum, pterygopalatine fossa to the floor of the orbit	Sensory	Skin of lower eyelid, cheeks and upper lip; mucosa of nasal cavity and sinuses; palate and upper teeth (infraorbital, zygomatic and superior alveolar branches)
V_c Mandibular	Foramen ovale, infratemporal fossa	Sensory	Skin of temple, cheek, chin, mucosa of inner cheek, anterior two-thirds of tongue and lower teeth (auriculotemporal, buccal, lingual, inferior alveolar and mental branches)
Small motor root	Foramen ovale, infratemporal fossa	Motor	Muscles of mastication (masseter, temporalis, medial and lateral pterygoids)
VI Abducent	Hindbrain junction between pons and medulla, cavernous sinus with internal carotid artery, superior orbital fissure, orbit	Motor	Extraocular muscle; lateral rectus

Table 3.56.1 (*cont'd*) THE 12 CRANIAL NERVES

Nerve	Origin, foramen and destination	Fibre types	Supply and function
VII Facial	Hindbrain between pons and medulla, internal auditory meatus: facial canal, stylomastoid foramen	Large motor root	Muscles of facial expression (temporal, zygomatic, buccal, mandibular and cervical branches), stapedius of middle ear, posterior belly of digastric
Nervus intermedius		Parasympathetic and special sensation	
	Greater petrosal nerve: passes via middle cranial fossa and pterygoid canal; neurones synapse in the pterygopalatine ganglion	Parasympathetic	Secretomotor to glands of nasal mucosa and sinuses, palate and lacrimal gland
	Chorda tympani: petrotympanic fissure behind temporomandibular joint; joins the lingual nerve V_3; neurones synapse in the submandibular ganglion	Parasympathetic	Secretomotor to the submandibular and sublingual glands
	Chorda tympani	Special sense	Taste from the anterior two-thirds of tongue
VIII Vestibulocochlear	Hindbrain cerebellopontine angle, internal auditory meatus (inner ear)	Special sense	Organs of balance and hearing (vestibular and cochlear branches)
IX Glossopharyngeal	Medulla, jugular foramen, pharynx	Mixed	
		Sensory	Meninges, pharyngeal sensation, carotid sinus (baroreceptor) and body (chemoreceptor), pharynx, middle ear
	Lesser petrosal passes upwards into the middle ear and middle cranial fossa; leaves cranium via the foramen ovale; neurones synapse in otic ganglion	Parasympathetic	Secretomotor to parotid gland
		Special sense	Taste to posterior one-third of tongue
X Vagus	Medulla, jugular foramen, neck (lies in carotid sheath), thorax and abdomen	Mixed	
		Sensory	Part of the external ear, external acoustic meatus and tympanic membrane, pharynx, larynx, visceral sensation from thorax and abdomen
		Motor	Intrinsic muscles of the larynx, pharynx, oesophagus; controls speech and swallowing
		Parasympathetic	Motor and secretomotor to thoracic and abdominal viscera
XI Accessory	Medulla gives rise to the cranial root; spinal root arises from spinal segments C1–C5; jugular foramen, posterior triangle of neck	Motor	
		Spinal root	Branchial muscles (trapezius and sternocleidomastoid)
		Cranial root	Joins with the vagus to supply pharynx and larynx
XII Hypoglossal	Medulla Hypoglossal canal Neck	Motor	Intrinsic and extrinsic muscles of the tongue; carries C_1 fibres that contribute to the anser cervicalis and supply the infrahyoid strap muscles

 DAMAGE TO THE SYMPATHETIC TRUNK

Horner's syndrome occurs if the sympathetic trunk is damaged as a result of trauma to the neck. Loss of the sympathetic supply to the head causes

- anhydrosis: loss of sweating on the face
- myosis: constriction of the pupil
- ptosis: drooping of the eyelid; the muscle that lifts the eyelid is partially smooth muscle (levator palpebrae superiores).

57. Major arteries

Questions
- Which two arteries supply the brain?
- What are the contents of the carotid sheath?
- Which part of the cranium is related to the middle meningeal artery?

Common carotid arteries

The right common carotid artery (CCA) arises from the brachiocephalic trunk behind the right sternoclavicular joint (Fig. 3.57.1). The left CCA arises directly from the aortic arch. The CCAs pass upwards on either side of the trachea, partially covered by the sternocleidomastoid muscle. The carotid pulse can be felt between this muscle and the larynx. The CCA, internal jugular vein and vagus nerve are enclosed by the carotid sheath. Posterior to the sheath is the cervical sympathetic chain. The CCA gives *no branches in the neck* and terminates at the upper border of the thyroid cartilage of the larynx (approximately C3) by dividing into the external and internal carotid arteries.

External carotid artery

The external corotid artery is anterior to both the internal jugular vein and internal carotid artery. It gives a number of branches that supply the neck, face and scalp. Level with the neck of the mandible, it enters the parotid gland and terminates as the maxillary and superficial temporal arteries. Its important branches are:

- **superior thyroid** anastomoses with the inferior thyroid from the subclavian to supply the thyroid and parathyroid glands, pharynx and larynx
- the superior laryngeal artery
- **lingual** loops around the hyoid and passes deep to hyoglossus to supply the tongue
- **facial** gives a branch to the palatine tonsils, makes an S bend around the submandibular gland before turning under the inferior border of the mandible onto the face; it passes superiorly to the medial corner of the eye
- **occipital and posterior auricular branches** supply the posterior scalp
- **superficial temporal** passes in front of the ear with the auriculotemporal nerve to supply the scalp
- **maxillary** supplies the muscles of mastication, upper and lower jaws and teeth and the nasal cavity; it also gives a branch to cranial cavity, the middle meningeal artery (Fig. 3.58.3).

Internal carotid artery

At the point of bifurcation of the CCA are the carotid sinuses, which monitor blood pressure (baroreceptors) and the carotid bodies (chemoreceptors); both are supplied by CN IX. The internal carotid has *no branches in the neck* and enters the base of the skull through the carotid canal, carrying a plexus of post-ganglionic sympathetic fibres. The canal is tortuous and passes medially before turning upwards. The artery makes an S-shaped turn as it lies within the cavernous sinus with CN VI and gives an ophthalmic branch before terminating as the anterior and middle cerebral arteries.

The ophthalmic artery divides with the orbit to supply the orbital contents and gives supraorbital and supratrochlear branches that supply the forehead and scalp. These branches anastomose with the superficial temporal artery. The most important orbital branch is the central artery of the retina (Fig. 3.67.1).

Vertebral arteries

The vertebral arteries (Fig. 3.57.2) arise from the first part of the subclavian artery. They pass upwards through the foramina transversaria of cervical vertebrae C_6 to C_1 to reach the foramen magnum, where they pierce the meninges and join on the anterior aspect of the pons to form the basilar artery. They supply the upper part of the spinal cord, the brainstem, cerebellum, posterior cerebral cortex and vestibular apparatus.

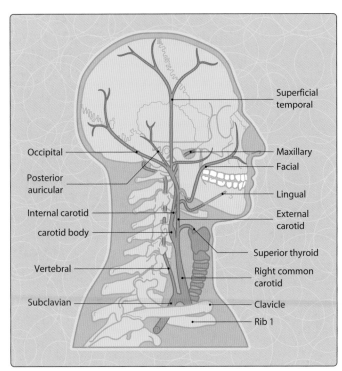

Occipital

Posterior auricular

Internal carotid

carotid body

Vertebral

Subclavian

Superficial temporal

Maxillary

Facial

Lingual

External carotid

Superior thyroid

Right common carotid

Clavicle

Rib 1

Fig. 3.57.1 Lateral view of the major arteries of the head and neck.

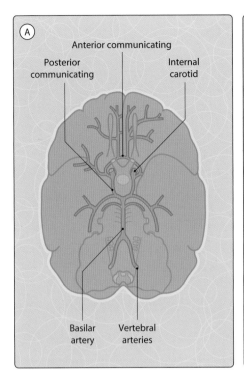

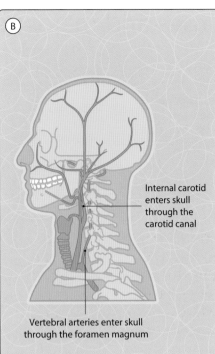

Fig. 3.57.2 The base of the brain. (A) View showing the vessels that form the circle of Willis; (B) lateral view showing the course of the vertebral arteries.

Anterior communicating

Posterior communicating

Internal carotid

Basilar artery

Vertebral arteries

Internal carotid enters skull through the carotid canal

Vertebral arteries enter skull through the foramen magnum

 CIRCLE OF WILLIS

The internal carotid and vertebral arteries supply the brain. They are connected by vessels that lie beneath the forebrain in the subarachnoid space (Fig. 3.57.2). The vertebral arteries join to form the basilar artery, which is connected via the posterior cerebral and posterior communicating branches with the internal carotid artery. The circle is completed by the anterior cerebral and anterior communicating branches. The precise arrangement is variable and the anastomosis may only be important if vessels are occluded by disease or blockage.

58. Dural venous sinuses and major veins

Questions
- How can infection spread from the central part of the face into the cranium?
- Why is it important to be able to locate the subclavian vein?

The major veins of the head and neck are shown in Fig. 3.58.1.

Dural venous sinuses

Blood from the brain drains to the dural venous sinuses (Figs 3.58.2–3.58.3).

The dural venous sinuses lie between the layers of the dura. They are lined by endothelium and there are no valves. They drain eventually to the internal jugular vein.

The **superior sagittal sinus** is enclosed in the superior margin of the falx cerebri (Fig. 3.55.2, p. 135) and drains posteriorly into the:

- right transverse sinus, lying along the lateral edge of the tentorium cerebelli
- right sigmoid sinus, which leaves the skull via the jugular foramen forming the right internal jugular vein.

The **inferior sagittal sinus** is enclosed in the inferior free margin of the falx cerebri and usually drains posteriorly into the:

- straight sinus, which also receives blood from the great cerebral vein

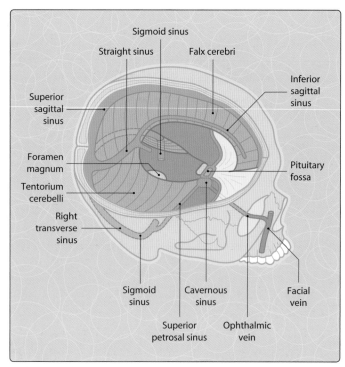

Fig. 3.58.2 View of the internal aspect of the cranium with the right side removed to show the relationship between the major dural venous sinuses, tentorium cerebelli and falx cerebri.

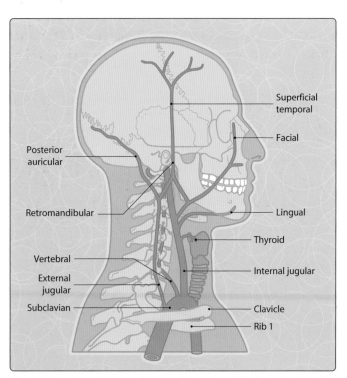

Fig. 3.58.1 Lateral view of the major veins of the head and neck.

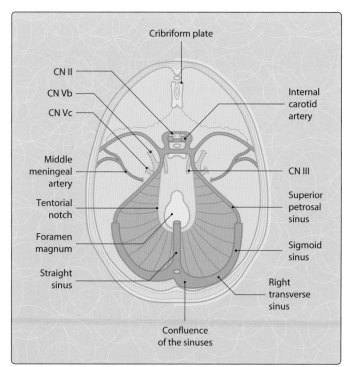

Fig. 3.58.3 View of the internal aspect of the cranium from above showing the tentorium cerebelli and associated dural venous sinuses.

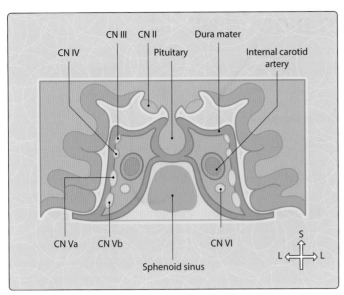

Fig. 3.58.4 Coronal section of the cavernous sinuses and pituitary gland.

- left transverse sinus
- left sigmoid sinus, which leaves the skull via the jugular foramen, forming the left internal jugular vein.

The **cavernous sinuses** (Figs 3.58.2–3.58.5) are complex venous channels lying on either side of the pituitary fossa that enclose the internal carotid artery and CN VI. They receive blood from ophthalmic veins and adjacent venous sinuses and then drain via the petrosal sinuses into the sigmoid sinuses on either side. Cranial nerves III, IV, V_a and V_b lie embedded in the dura of the lateral wall of the cavernous sinus (Fig. 3.58.4). Because the cavernous sinuses are connected with the face via the ophthalmic veins, it is possible for infections to spread centrally, which may result in thrombosis and sepsis. Such an infection affects the cranial nerves associated with the cavernous sinuses and blockage of the venous drainage of the orbit.

Internal jugular vein

The internal jugular vein is a large vessel that begins as the continuation of the sigmoid sinus at the margins of the jugular foramen and lies deep to sternocleidomastoid throughout its course in the neck (Fig. 3.58.1). It ends by joining with the subclavian vein to form the brachiocephalic vein. On the left,

this junction is the point at which the **thoracic duct** returns lymph to the venous system (Fig. 3.66.2, p. 156). On the right is the smaller right lymphatic duct. The brachiocephalic veins join to form the superior vena cava. The internal jugular receives veins that accompany the arterial branches of the external carotid artery.

External jugular vein

The **maxillary** and **superficial temporal veins** join together in the substance of the parotid gland (p. 143) forming the **retromandibular vein** (its name tells you where it lies). As the retromandibular vein leaves the parotid gland, it divides into anterior and posterior divisions. The posterior auricular and posterior divisions of the retromandibular vein join to form the **external jugular,** which empties into the subclavian vein. The anterior jugular vein begins below the chin and runs close to the midline before also draining into the external jugular vein.

The **facial vein** accompanies the artery as it crosses the face and drains with the anterior division of the retromandibular vein into the external jugular vein (Fig. 3.58.1). The facial veins are connected to the intracranial dural venous sinuses via the ophthalmic veins (Fig. 3.58.2).

Subclavian vein

The upper limb is drained by the **subclavian vein**. It receives the external jugular vein, and veins corresponding to the branches of the subclavian artery, eventually joining with the internal jugular to form the brachiocephalic vein behind the sterno-clavicular joint. The subclavian vein is the most anterior structure lying on the first rib just behind the middle of the clavicle; it is an important site of venous access (central venous line, p. 67).

 JUGULAR VENOUS PRESSURE

The external jugular vein is often visible, lying superficial to the sternocleidomastoid muscle. It is observed clinically when assessing jugular venous pressure. Pulsations of the vein are normally seen at the level of the jugular notch; however, in heart failure, pulsations will reach a higher level.

59. Scalp, face, facial nerve and parotid gland

Questions
- Which cranial nerve supplies the skin of the face?
- What is the nerve supply to the muscles of facial expression?
- Disease of which salivary gland is likely to affect the way you smile?

Scalp

The scalp receives a very good blood supply from anastomosing branches of the internal and external carotid arteries. It is for this reason that we lose a great deal of heat from the head and why scalp and facial wounds bleed freely and heal quickly. Anteriorly, its sensory nerve supply comes from CN V, laterally and posteriorly from C_2 (Fig. 3.59.1). It comprises a series of layers, which are illustrated in Fig. 3.55.1 (p. 135).

Face

Cutaneous nerve supply

Skin sensation of the face is supplied entirely by branches of the trigeminal nerve (Fig. 3.59.1). A small area over the angle of the jaw and the lower part of the parotid gland are supplied by the **great auricular nerve** (from the cervical plexus). The concavity opposite to the tragus of the external ear is supplied by the

vagus nerve and pain from the motor distribution of the vagus (e.g. larynx, pharynx) may be referred to the ear.

Facial artery

The **facial artery** is a branch of the external carotid artery (Fig. 3.57.1, p. 138). It crosses the lower border of the mandible at the anterior edge of masseter (where its pulse can be felt). It supplies the upper and lower lips and ends at the inner corner of the eye. The facial vein accompanies the artery.

Facial nerve and the muscles of facial expression

The muscles of facial expression are supplied by the facial nerve CN VII (Fig. 3.59.2 and Table 3.59.1). Muscles that act as dilators and sphincters are arranged around the eyes, nose and mouth; the major muscles are listed in the table. They insert into the skin and their actions give expression to human emotions. Paralysis of these muscles can be a devastating disability.

The parotid gland

The facial nerve emerges from the skull close to the mastoid process and passes into the parotid gland, where it lies very superficially and divides to form a plexus. Its branches emerge from the anterior margin of the parotid gland (Fig. 3.59.3). Remember that diseases of the parotid may affect CN VII.

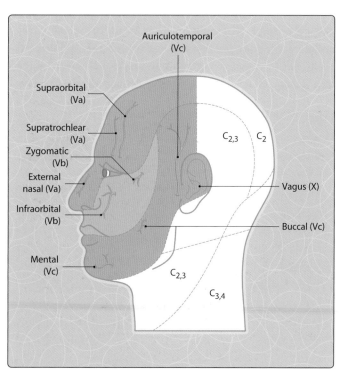

Fig. 3.59.1 Lateral view of the head showing the distribution of the cutaneous branches of the trigeminal nerve.

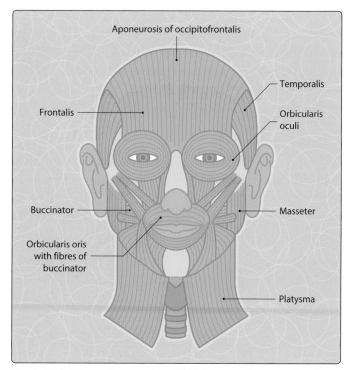

Fig. 3.59.2 The major muscles of facial expression, anterior view.

Table 3.59.1 MUSCLES OF FACIAL EXPRESSION

Branch of VII	Muscles	
Temporal	Frontal belly of occipitofrontalis	Raises the eyebrows
	Orbicularis oculi	Blinking the upper eyelid
Zygomatic	Orbicularis oculi	Blinking the lower eyelid
Buccal	Buccinator	Pushes food from the vestibule of the mouth to the oral cavity
	Orbicularis oris	Moves the upper lip
Marginal mandibular	Orbicularis oris	Moves the lower lip
Cervical	Platysma	Pulls down the angle of the mouth

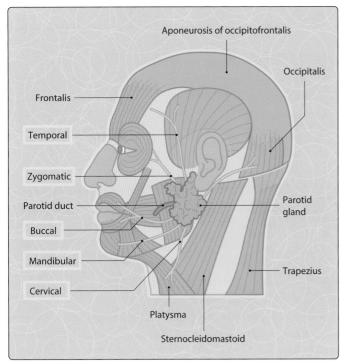

Fig. 3.59.3 Lateral view of the muscles of facial expression, the parotid gland and the branches of the facial nerve.

The parotid gland is a large salivary gland that lies wedged between the angle of the mandible and the mastoid process (Fig. 3.59.4). Its duct emerges from the anterior border, crosses the masseter muscle and pierces buccinator, opening into the vestibule of the mouth opposite the second molar tooth. The retromandibular vein, auriculotemporal nerve and the terminal part of the external carotid artery all pass through the gland. It is supplied by parasympathetic nerves that travel in the lesser petrosal branch of CN IX, synapse in the otic ganglion and are distributed by the auriculotemporal nerve. Infection of the gland leads to the swelling known as mumps.

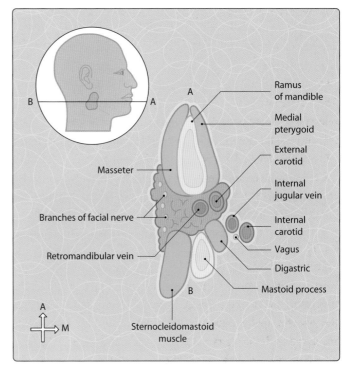

Fig. 3.59.4 Transverse section through the parotid gland and associated structures.

 APPLIED ANATOMY OF THE SCALP

A useful acronym is SCALP:
- <u>s</u>kin: numerous hair follicles and associated glands are prone to sebaceous cyst formation
- <u>c</u>onnective tissue: contains cutaneous nerves and blood vessels; septa divide the layer into compartments, making it tricky to give *effective* injections of local anaesthetic
- <u>a</u>poneurosis: the tendon connects frontalis anteriorly and occipitalis posteriorly; transverse lacerations will gape because of the pull of the aponeurosis and black eye may develop after a blow to the top of the head because blood can track under the aponeurosis to the face (subaponeurotic haematoma)
- <u>l</u>oose areolar tissue: the three superficial layers are tightly bound together allowing them to move freely in this plane
- <u>p</u>ericranium (the periosteum of the skull): forceps delivery of a child may result in subperiosteal bleeding that is limited by the attachment of the pericranium at the suture joints; therefore, the area of bleeding matches the shape of the bones (cephalohaematoma).

60. Temporomandibular joint and mastication

Questions
- Which cranial nerve supplies all the muscles of mastication?
- What muscle brings about protraction of the mandible?
- What is the importance of the middle meningeal artery?

Mastication

There are four muscles of mastication; all are supplied by the motor root of CN V.

- **Masseter** (Fig. 3.60.1) lies in the cheek. Clench your teeth and feel the muscle as it contracts in your cheek down to the angle of your jaw; it elevates the mandible.
- **Temporalis** occurs over the temple (its posterior fibres also retract the jaw); clench your teeth and feel it contract over your temple (elevator) (Fig. 3.60.2).
- The **lateral and medial pterygoids** (Fig. 3.60.3) lie deep to the ramus of the mandible in the infratemporal fossa. By contracting alternately, they produce the side-to-side movements of the mandible as food is chewed; the lateral pterygoid also brings about the protraction required in wide opening of the mouth.

The buccinator is a muscle of facial expression and is supplied by CN VII; however, it assists chewing. The **buccinator** (Fig. 3.60.1) forms the lateral walls of the mouth (cheek); anteriorly some of its fibres merge with orbicularis oris and posteriorly it forms a raphe with the superior constrictor of the

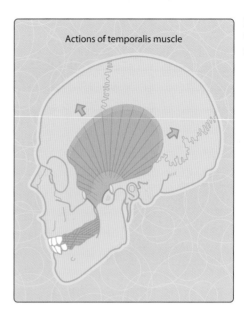

Fig. 3.60.2 Lateral view of temporalis muscle.

Actions of temporalis muscle

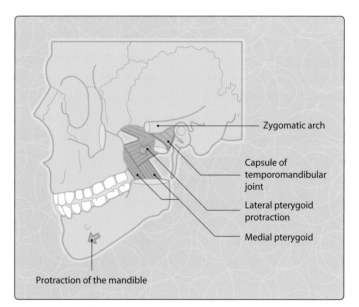

- Zygomatic arch
- Capsule of temporomandibular joint
- Lateral pterygoid protraction
- Medial pterygoid

Protraction of the mandible

Fig. 3.60.3 Lateral view of the infratemporal fossa showing the pterygoid muscles (zygomatic arch and part of the ramus of the mandible removed).

pharynx (Fig. 3.63.1, p. 150). It assists chewing by forcing food from the vestibule (between the cheek and molar teeth) back towards the oral cavity.

Temporomandibular joint

Movements of mastication take place at the temporomandibular joint. A large, fibrocartilagenous disc (Fig. 3.60.4) divides the cavity into two separate compartments. During small movements (talking), the disc is stationary and the head of the

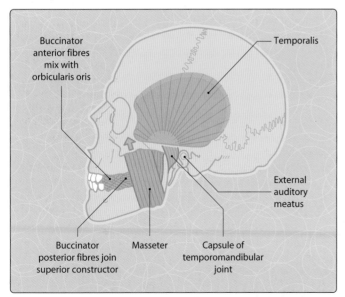

Buccinator anterior fibres mix with orbicularis oris

Temporalis

External auditory meatus

Buccinator posterior fibres join superior constrictor

Masseter

Capsule of temporomandibular joint

Fig. 3.60.1 Lateral view of the superficial muscles of mastication showing the action of masseter.

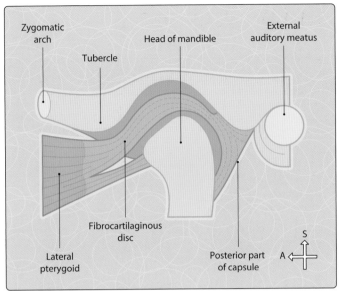

Zygomatic arch

Tubercle

Head of mandible

External auditory meatus

Lateral pterygoid

Fibrocartilaginous disc

Posterior part of capsule

S
A

Fig. 3.60.4 Sagittal section of the temporomandibular joint showing the intra-articular disc.

mandible moves within the concavity of the disc (Fig. 3.60.5A). When the mouth is opened widely (depression and protraction of the jaw), the lateral pterygoid muscles pull the head of the mandible and the disc forwards together so that the disc moves across the articular surface of the temporal bone (Fig. 3.60.5B). You can feel this movement of the mandibular head by placing a finger just in front of your ear as you open your mouth widely. Small depression movements do not involve protraction; they are caused by digastric and mylohyoid assisted by gravity. Because the joint is supplied by the auriculotemporal nerve, a branch of V_c (Fig. 3.59.1, p. 142), pain from the temporomandibular joint can be referred to the external ear.

Infratemporal fossa

The infratemporal fossa is the space deep to the ramus of the

mandible in front of and beneath the temporal bone; it contains muscles, arteries, veins and nerves and their relations are complex.

- **Muscles.** The lateral and medial pterygoid muscles act upon the temporomandibular joint to depress and protract the mandible.
- The **terminal branches** of the **external carotid artery**. Behind the ramus of the mandible, the external carotid divides to form the maxillary and superficial temporal arteries. The maxillary artery branches extensively within the fossa, but its most important branch is the **middle meningeal artery** (see below). The pulse of the superficial temporal artery can be felt in front of the ear; it supplies the scalp and is accompanied by the auriculotemporal nerve.
- The **mandibular nerve** comprises sensory fibres of V_c and the motor root of V (p. 136). It enters the infratemporal fossa through the foramen ovale. It branches to supply the muscles of mastication (e.g. masseter, temporalis), the mandible and lower teeth (inferior alveolar nerve), the tongue (lingual nerve), skin of the cheek (buccal nerve) and scalp (auriculotemporal nerve).
- The **pterygoid venous plexus**. This network of veins forms interconnections between facial and ophthalmic veins with the dural venous sinuses, particularly the cavernous sinus.

EXTRADURAL HAEMORRHAGE

The **middle meningeal artery** arises from the maxillary artery and passes upwards, *via* the foramen spinosum into the middle cranial fossa, where it supplies the meninges and diploë of the skull. Within the skull, it lies in direct contact with the cranium, grooving the bone. It is very vulnerable in fractures of the **pterion** (the thinnest region of the skull), where a blow to the head may cause an extradural haemorrhage (p. 132).

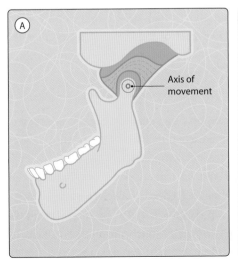

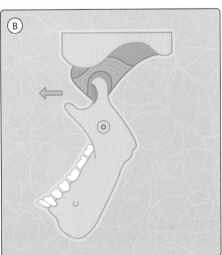

Ⓐ

Axis of movement

Ⓑ

Fig. 3.60.5 Sagittal sections of the temporomandibular joint showing the axis of rotation in (A) small movements of the jaw (disc stationary) and (B) wide opening of the jaw (disc and head are pulled anteriorly by the lateral pterygoid (attachment in red)).

61. Orbit

Questions
- Which three cranial nerves supply the extraocular muscles?
- Which cranial nerve has the longest intracranial course?
- Which nerve controls blinking of the eyelids?

Eyelids

The eyelids are stiffened by rigid **tarsal plates** (Figs 3.61.1 and 3.61.2); these are covered in front by loose skin and the circularly arranged muscle fibres of **orbicularis oculi**, which bring about blinking (Fig. 3.59.2). The **levator palpebrae superioris** is antagonistic to the action of orbicularis oculi, lifting the upper eyelid. It is partly formed from smooth muscle supplied by sympathetic nerves, damage to which leads to drooping of the eyelid (ptosis). The 'buttonhole' opening between the lids is the **palpebral fissure**. The **conjunctiva** protects the exposed surface of the cornea and lines the undersurface of the eyelids to form the conjunctival sacs. **Tarsal glands** produce an oily secretion that delays evaporation of tears from the surface of the conjunctiva (Fig. 3.61.2).

Lacrimal apparatus

Tucked into the upper lateral corner of the orbits are the **lacrimal glands** (Fig. 3.61.1), which continuously secrete tears into the superior fornix of the conjunctival sac (Fig. 3.61.2). Normal reflex blinking spreads tears across the eyeball from

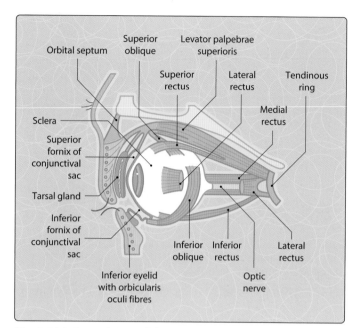

Fig. 3.61.2 Lateral view of the eyelid, eyeball and cone of extraocular muscles.

lateral to medial; any excess drains via the **lacrimal puncta and canaliculi** into the **nasolacrimal sac** and **duct,** which opens into the inferior meatus of the nasal cavity (Fig. 3.64.1). The glands receive a secretomotor supply from postganglionic parasympathetic neurons, which travel in the greater petrosal nerve of CN VII and synapse in the pterygopalatine ganglion before hitchhiking with the zygomatic branch of CN V_b and the lacrimal branch of CN V_a.

The orbit

The orbit contains the eyeball (p. 158), optic nerve and extraocular muscles and supports the eyelids and lacrimal apparatus. The ophthalmic artery and the cranial nerves that supply these structures and the upper part of the face and scalp enter the orbit through the optic canal and superior and inferior orbital fissures (Fig. 3.61.3).

Extraocular muscles

The eyeball is supported by a **suspensory ligament** attached to either side of the orbit like a hammock (Figs 3.61.1 and 3.61.4) so contraction of the extraocular muscles can swivel the eyeballs around their vertical and horizontal axes, coordinating their gaze to a single point; failure leads to double vision (Fig. 3.61.5).

The four recti muscles are attached to a tendinous ring at the back of the orbit and form a cone around the eyeball by attaching to the sclera just behind the cornea (Figs 3.61.2–3.61.4).

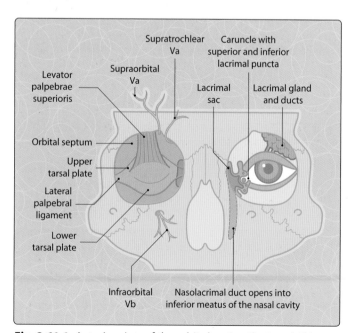

Fig. 3.61.1 Anterior view of the orbit showing the tarsal plates and levator palpebrae superioris (left) and the lacrimal apparatus (right).

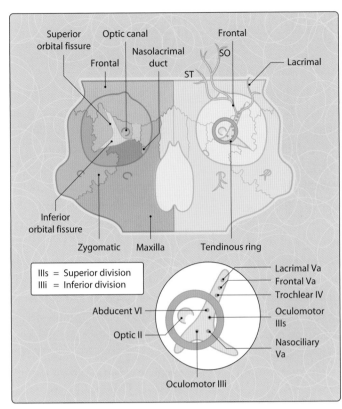

Fig. 3.61.3 Anterior view showing the osteology of the orbit (left) and the position of the tendinous ring (right). Inset shows the details of the nerves entering the orbit through the superior orbital fissure.

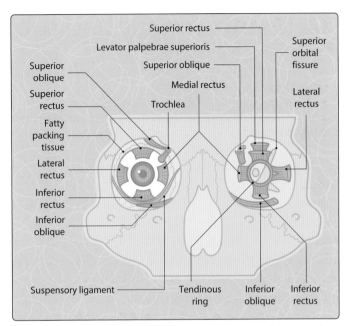

Fig. 3.61.4 Anterior view of the orbit showing attachments of the extraocular muscles (left) and the position of the tendinous ring, posterior foramina and cranial nerves, visible when the eyeball is removed (right).

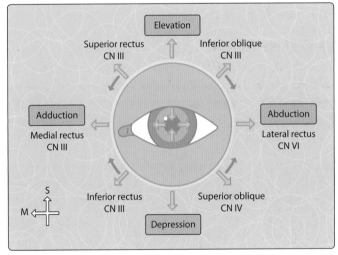

Fig. 3.61.5 Diagram to show the action and nerve supply of the extraocular muscles. Arrows show the direction that the pupil moves when muscle action occurs.

The two **oblique muscles** reach the eyeball from the bony wall of the orbit. The superior oblique arises in the posterior part of the orbit and hooks round a pulley or **trochlea** in the medial corner of the orbit. It is supplied by the **trochlear nerve** (CN IV), which has the longest intracranial course of all the cranial nerves and is, therefore, often the first nerve to be affected in raised intracranial pressure. The inferior oblique arises in the anteromedial corner of the orbit.

Oculomotor nerve

The oculomotor nerve (CN III) pierces the roof of the cavernous sinus and passes anteriorly embedded in the wall of the sinus (Fig. 3.58.4, p. 141). It enters the orbit through the superior orbital fissure and carries preganglionic parasympathetic fibres, which synapse in the ciliary ganglion and supply the constrictor pupillae and ciliary body. The dilator pupillae is supplied by sympathetic fibres from the superior cervical ganglion; these fibres accompany the internal carotid and ophthalmic arteries and eventually the nasociliary branch of CN V$_a$.

 THE OCULOMOTOR NERVE

The oculomotor nerve, CN III, may be stretched and damaged if the pressure within the cranium increases (e.g. in intracranial bleeding), affecting five of the extraocular muscles and the ciliary body. Damage causes:

- ptosis (loss of motor supply to levator palpebrae superioris)
- lateral squint (all extraocular muscles are paralysed except superior oblique and lateral rectus)
- dilatation of pupil (sympathetic supply to pupil is unopposed)
- loss of accommodation and light reflexes.

62. Mouth, tongue and submandibular region

Questions
- Which cranial nerve supplies the muscles of the tongue?
- What is the sensory nerve supply of the anterior two-thirds of the tongue?

Mouth

The mouth extends from the lips to the **palatoglossal fold** immediately anterior to the **tonsils** (Fig. 3.62.1). The roof is formed by the **hard palate** anteriorly (maxilla and palatine bones) and posteriorly by the **soft palate** and uvula (muscular). The palatoglossal fold, soft palate and the dorsal surface of the tongue form the oropharyngeal isthmus, separating the mouth from the oropharynx. The mouth has two parts: the **vestibule** between the cheeks (forming the lateral walls) and teeth and the **oral cavity** internal to the teeth (Fig. 3.62.2). The teeth are embedded in the gums (gingivae) covering the inferior and superior alveolar processes. The floor is formed by the tongue and the mylohyoid muscle (Fig. 3.62.3).

Tongue

The tongue consists of striated muscle covered by a stratified squamous epithelium with many small salivary glands. Its movements are complex and important in speech, chewing, suckling and swallowing. It is attached to the floor of the mouth by the **frenulum**.

Arterial and nerve supply

The dorsum of the tongue is studded with papillae many of which are associated with taste buds. It is divided into an anterior oral two-thirds and a posterior pharyngeal one-third by the V-shaped **sulcus terminalis** with the **foramen caecum** at its apex (Fig. 3.62.1). Immediately anterior to the sulcus are 7–12 **vallate papillae**. Posteriorly, the tongue is smooth with raised nodules of lymphoid tissue, which form the **lingual tonsil**.

The tongue has a rich blood supply from the lingual artery, and venous drainage is to the internal jugular vein. Deep veins are visible on the undersurface. The tongue is commonly affected by cancer so it is important to understand its lymphatic drainage. The tip drains to the submental nodes and the rest to the submandibular and deep cervical nodes. Lymph drains across the median septum particularly posteriorly and may lead to bilateral spread of cancer.

The oral two-thirds of the tongue receives common sensory innervation from the lingual nerve (CN V_c) with taste fibres from the chorda tympani (p. 137). The pharyngeal one-third, including the vallate papillae, is innervated by the pharyngeal plexus (CN IX and X).

Submandibular and sublingual glands

The submandibular gland lies beneath and medial to the angle of the mandible, with the lingual artery curving around it. It is deeply indented by the mylohyoid muscle, which divides it into

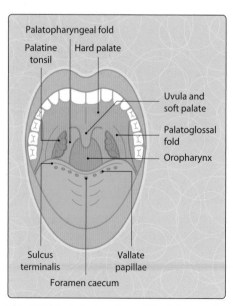

Fig. 3.62.1 Anterior view of the interior of the oral cavity.

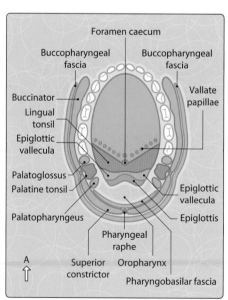

Fig. 3.62.2 Horizontal section of the mouth showing the cheeks, dorsum of the tongue and oropharynx.

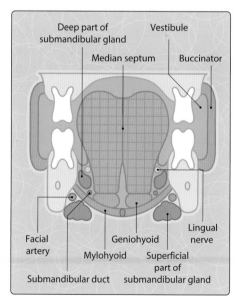

Fig. 3.62.3 Coronal section of the mouth showing the posterior part of the submandibular region opposite the third molar tooth.

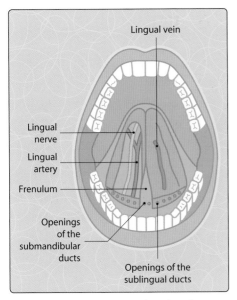

Fig. 3.62.4 Anterior view showing the undersurface of the tongue.

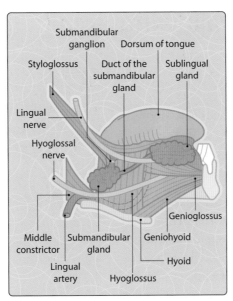

Fig. 3.62.5 Lateral view of the tongue, mandible removed, to show the submandibular gland and duct.

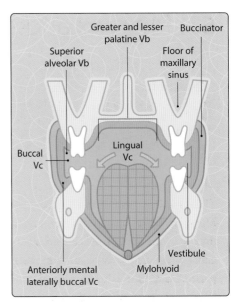

Fig. 3.62.6 Coronal section of the mouth showing the nerve supply of the oral mucosa.

Table 3.62.1 MUSCLES AND MOVEMENTS OF THE TONGUE

Muscle	Attachments	Nerve supply	Action
Intrinsic muscles	Longitudinal, transverse and vertical groups	CN XII (hypoglossal) supplies all except palatoglossus	Change shape of the tongue
Extrinsic muscles			Depression
1 Hyoglossus	Hyoid bone (below and lateral)		Depression and protrusion
2 Genioglossus	Inside the anterior part of mandible (below)		Pulls the posterior tongue
3 Styloglossus	Styloid process (above and lateral)		up and back during swallowing
			Closure of the oropharyngeal
4 Palatoglossus	Palate (above)	CN IX	isthmus during swallowing

superficial and deep parts. The duct passes forward close to the lingual nerve and opens alongside the frenulum (Figs 3.62.3–3.62.5). The duct is prone to blockage with stones. The **sublingual glands** are the smallest of the three major salivary glands. They are scattered along the submandibular duct and open along the sublingual folds at the base of the frenulum.

Both glands receive a parasympathetic secretomotor supply by way of chorda tympani fibres (CN VII) carried by the lingual nerve and synapsing in the submandibular ganglion (Fig. 3.62.6).

63. Pharynx and swallowing

Questions
- Which nerves make up the pharyngeal plexus?
- How may infection spread from the nasopharynx to the middle ear?
- Which structures lie anterior and posterior to the palatine tonsils?

The pharynx lies posterior to the nose, mouth and larynx, forming the upper portions of the digestive and respiratory tracts. It is not a complete tube as it has no proper anterior wall. It consists of superior, middle and inferior constrictor muscles (Figs 3.63.1 and 3.63.2), which are stacked inside each other like paper cups. The muscle fibres pass inferiorly and laterally from a posterior line of fusion (raphe) to attach to their various anterior bony insertions (Fig. 3.63.2):

- **superior constrictor** merges with the posterior fibres of buccinator to form the cheeks (Fig. 3.60.1, p. 144)
- **middle constrictor** is attached partly to the hyoid bone
- **inferior constrictor** attaches to the thyroid and cricoid cartilages of the larynx.

The constrictors are lined internally by pharyngobasilar fascia and the mucosa of the pharynx (Fig. 3.62.2). There are also three longitudinal muscles that lift the pharynx during swallowing.

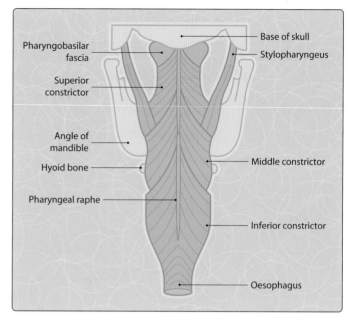

Fig. 3.63.2 Posterior view of the constrictor muscles of the pharynx.

The pharynx has three subdivisions: naso-, oro- and laryngopharynx (Figs 3.63.3–3.63.6). The **nasopharynx** lies between the posterior nasal aperture and the pharyngeal isthmus at the level of the soft palate; it contains:

- opening of the **auditory (Eustachian) tube**, allowing equalization of air pressure between the nasopharynx and the middle ear cavity (also a route for the spread infection)
- **tubal tonsil** (lymphoid tissue) surrounds the opening of the auditory tubes; inflammation may cause blockage
- **nasopharyngeal tonsil** on the posterior wall ('adenoids').

The **oropharynx** lies behind the mouth between the pharyngeal isthmus and epiglottis. Anteriorly, the palatoglossal fold forms the oropharyngeal isthmus. The posterior wall is formed by superior constrictor muscle, lying anterior to atlas and axis vertebrae. The **palatine tonsils** lie between palatoglossal and palatopharyngeal folds (anterior and posterior pillars of fauces; Fig. 3.62.2). The palatine, tubal, naospharyngeal and lingual tonsils form Waldeyer's ring of subepithelial lymphoid tissue, which is particularly obvious in children.

The **laryngopharynx** is the common passage for the digestive and respiratory tracts. It lies between the epiglottis and the beginning of the oesophagus at C6 (Fig. 3.63.4). The most inferior part acts as a sphincter to control entry to the oesophagus. On either side of the laryngeal inlet are the **piriform fossae,** which channel food and fluids laterally, bypassing the laryngeal opening. Posterior to the tongue, the median and lateral glosso-

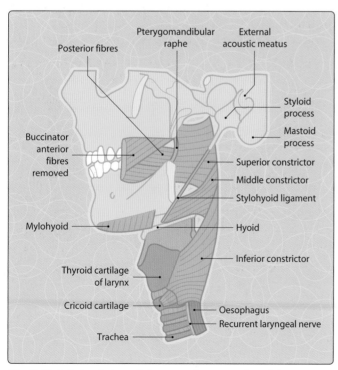

Fig. 3.63.1 Lateral view of the constrictor muscles of the pharynx; ramus of the mandible and zygomatic arch removed.

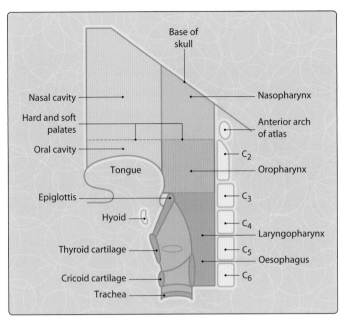

Fig. 3.63.3 The subdivisions of the pharynx.

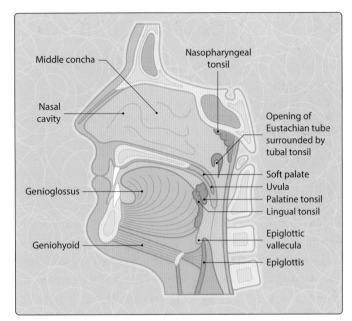

Fig. 3.63.5 Median section of the head to show the internal features of the nasal cavity and pharynx.

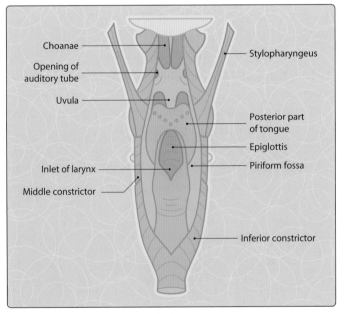

Fig. 3.63.4 Posterior view with the constrictors opened.

epiglottic folds form the **epiglottic valleculae,** where foreign bodies may become lodged (Fig. 3.62.2).

Blood, nerve and lymphatic systems

Nerve supply is from the pharyngeal plexus: CN IX (sensory–gag reflex), CN X and cranial fibres of CN XI (motor supply to striated muscle), sympathetic (vasoconstrictor).

During swallowing:

- the tongue lifts, forcing food into the posterior third of the oral cavity (CN XII)
- the Eustachian tube opens (CN X)
- the soft palate closes the pharyngeal isthmus, preventing food passing into the nasopharynx (CN X)
- the oropharyngeal isthmus is closed to prevent reflux into the mouth (CN IX)
- the laryngeal inlet is reduced in size to prevent passage of food into the larynx (CN X)
- the larynx is raised towards the hyoid and the base of the tongue (CN VII, CN IX, CN X)
- the epiglottis flips down to cover the laryngeal inlet.

Blood supply is from local branches of the external carotid, draining to internal and external jugular veins. Lymphatic drainage is to the deep cervical and retropharyngeal nodes.

64. Nose, paranasal air sinuses and larynx

Questions
- Which bones form the lateral wall of the nasal cavity?
- What type of epithelium lines the paranasal air sinuses?
- What is the nerve supply to muscles of the larynx?

Nose

The nose is the upper part of the airway and is continuous via the naso- and oropharynx with the larynx and trachea. The external nose consists of the **nasal bones** and a mobile part composed of fibrocartilage. The skin is supplied by the external nasal nerve (CN V_a). The anterior openings of the nose are the nostrils (nares) divided by the **nasal septum** (Fig. 3.64.1). The **nasal cavities** extend from the nostrils to the choanae posteriorly and are continuous with the nasopharynx (see Ch. 63); they are bordered by:

- **lateral wall:** maxilla, ethmoid and three conchae (superior, middle and inferior) and palatine bones; the area inferior to each of the conchae is the equivalent **meatus**
- **nasal septum:** a posterior bony portion (ethmoid and vomer) and a large anterior septal cartilage; the septum rarely lies exactly in the midline
- **floor:** hard palate (maxilla and palatine)
- **roof:** cribriform plate through which pass the branches of CN I (olfaction).

The upper one-third of the nasal cavity is innervated by branches of CN V_a and supplied by branches of the ophthalmic artery while the lower two-thirds is innervated by branches of CN V_b and supplied by branches of the maxillary artery. The nasal cavity and paranasal sinuses are lined by respiratory epithelium.

Paranasal air sinuses

The frontal, maxillary and ethmoidal sinuses are paired; the sphenoidal sinus lies in the midline anterior to the pituitary gland. The lowest part of the **maxillary sinus** lies at the level of the roots of the maxillary teeth. Because the opening into the nasal cavity is high on the medial wall of the sinus, mucus may be trapped, become infected and result in sinusitis (Fig. 3.64.1C).

Larynx

You need to understand the anatomy of the larynx to perform intubation of the airway in an unconscious patient and to understand its appearance using a laryngoscope (Fig. 3.68.1). The larynx consists of a series of hyaline cartilages connected by fibroelastic membranes and muscles that move the cartilages (Fig. 3.64.2). In an emergency when the larynx becomes blocked by a foreign body or by swelling, a hollow needle may be inserted into the cricothyroid membrane just below the thyroid prominence.

The internal aspect of the larynx is lined by mucous membrane. The **vocal cords** or folds are formed where the membrane folds over two fibrous bands that stretch from the arytenoid cartilages behind to the thyroid cartilage in front (Fig. 3.64.3). The cords lie together at the level of C_4 (just below

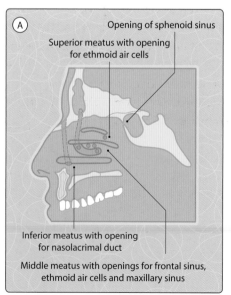

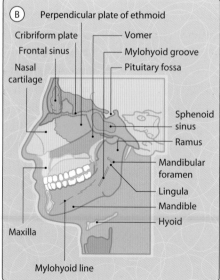

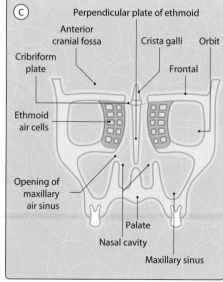

Fig. 3.64.1 The face and nasal cavity. (A) Lateral view showing nasal septum and medial features of the mandible; (B) removal of conchae reveals the openings of the paranasal air sinuses; (C) coronal section shows the ethmoid bone.

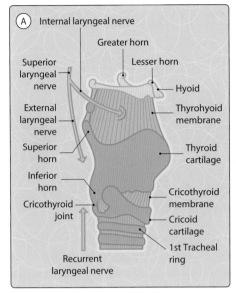
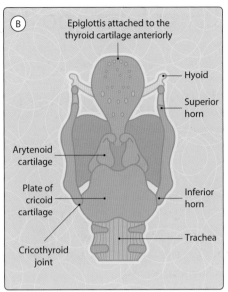
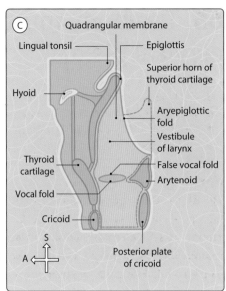

Fig. 3.64.2 Laryngeal cartilages and membranes. (A) Lateral view; (B) posterior view; (C) median section.

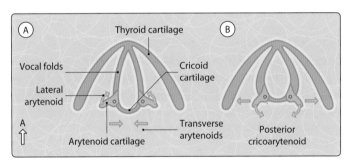

Fig. 3.64.3 Transverse section through the larynx at the level of the vocal folds to show the movements of the arytenoid cartilages. (A) Adduction (action of the lateral arytenoid and transverse arytenoid muscles); (B) abduction and rotation (action of the posterior cricothyroid muscle).

the laryngeal prominence) and with the arytenoid cartilages form the **glottis**. Immediately above the true vocal folds are **false vocal folds,** which lie at the inferior margin of the vestibule.

The larynx performs three major functions.

1. *Phonation.* Oscillations in the air passing between the vocal cords produce a buzz, which is modified by the mouth, lips and tongue to produce speech. Movement at the cricothyroid joint increases the *tension* of the vocal folds and raises the pitch of the voice.

2. *Control of the glottic aperture.* Rotation and/or abduction of the arytenoid cartilages enlarges the shape of the glottis, allowing an increase in air intake (Fig. 3.64.3).

3. *Control of the inlet during swallowing.* The aryepiglottic folds contract like a sphincter to help to close the inlet.

Blood and nerve supply

Blood supply to the larynx is from the superior thyroid artery; venous drainage is to the internal and external jugular veins and lymphatic drainage is to the deep cervical chain.

Innervation of the larynx is described on p. 157:

- sensory above the vocal cords: superior laryngeal CN X
- sensory below the vocal cords (subglottal): recurrent laryngeal CN X
- motor laryngeal muscles: recurrent laryngeal CN X.

Disease of the larynx may result in referred pain to the external ear because both are supplied by the vagus nerve.

65. The bony muscular column, posterior triangle and cervical plexus

Questions
- What layer of fascia binds the thyroid gland to the trachea?
- What are the contents of the carotid sheath?
- What is the most important motor branch of the cervical plexus?

The neck supports the head and provides attachments for the muscles that move the head and the neck (Fig. 3.65.1). The fascial layers in the neck allow free movement of adjacent structures and are important in the spread of disease. The neck initially seems complex, but it is useful to think of it consisting of five columns (Fig. 3.65.2).

Column 1: bony muscular column.   This column is enclosed by **prevertebral fascia**, which covers the prevertebral and scalene muscles into the thorax. The tissue space between the prevertebral fascia and the pharynx/oesophagus (**retropharyngeal space**) allows infections to track from the pharynx to the mediastinum. The cervical sympathetic trunk lies here, immediately posterior to the carotid sheath.

Column 2: visceral column.   This is a column comprising pharynx/oesophagus, larynx/trachea and the thyroid gland.

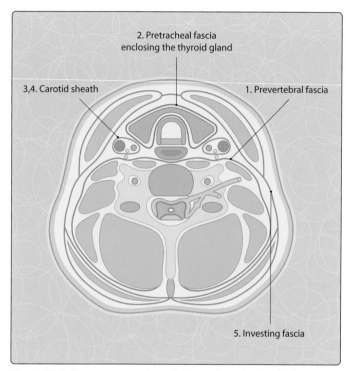

Fig. 3.65.2 Transverse section of the neck at the level of C_6 to show the fascial planes and the five columns described in the text.

It is enclosed by **pretracheal fascia**, which extends from the thyroid cartilage above to the fibrous pericardium below.

Columns 3 and 4: two neurovascular bundles.   These are surrounded by the **carotid sheath,** which forms a tube surrounding the common and internal carotid arteries, internal jugular vein, vagus nerve between them and the cervical chain of lymph nodes. The carotid sheath is attached superiorly to the margins of the carotid canal in the base of skull and blends inferiorly with the aortic arch.

Column 5: the whole neck.   The final column is the whole neck itself, enclosed by **deep investing fascia**, which wraps around it like a collar. The fascia splits to enclose trapezius, sternocleidomastoid, the strap muscles and the parotid and submandibular glands. It is attached superiorly to the base of the skull, inferiorly to the bones of the pectoral girdle and posteriorly to the nuchal ligament.

The bony muscular column

The cervical spine consists of seven vertebrae (p. 28). Because it is the most mobile region of the vertebral column, the intervertebral joints are prone to wear and tear, causing pain through irritation of cervical spinal nerves (remember that C_4–C_7 are

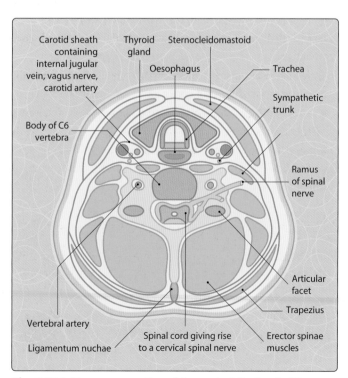

Fig. 3.65.1 Transverse section of the neck at the level of C_6.

distributed to the upper limb by branches of the brachial plexus). Muscular action involves:

- **postvertebral muscles** bring about extension against gravity, e.g. erector spinae and suboccipital muscles (supplied segmentally by the *dorsal* rami of cervical nerves)
- **prevertebral** and **lateral muscles** bring about flexion and lateral flexion and are separated from the pharynx anteriorly by prevertebral fascia, e.g. scalene muscles (supplied segmentally by the *ventral* rami of cervical nerves).

Posterior triangle of the neck

Figure 3.65.3 shows the contents of the posterior triangle of the neck. Its **boundaries are**:

- anterior   posterior border of sternocleidomastoid muscle
- posterior   anterior border of trapezius
- inferior   middle part of the clavicle.

Crossing the triangle are the **supraclavicular nerves** and the **external jugular vein** (Fig. 3.65.3 and p. 140).

The contents of the posterior triangle are:

- trunks of the brachial plexus
- apex of the lung, extending 2.5 cm above the middle one-third of the clavicle (Fig. 3.66.2)
- spinal part of the accessory nerve CN XI
- cervical plexus C_1–C_4 (Fig. 3.65.4)
- lymph nodes (p. 157)
- subclavian artery: divided into three parts.

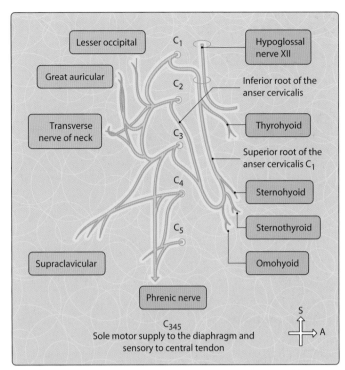

Fig. 3.65.4 Lateral view of the cervical plexus showing the distribution of the motor (blue) and sensory (pink) branches. Motor supply is to the infrahyoid muscles and diaphragm; sensory branches come from the skin of the neck.

Subclavian artery

The subclavian artery is a short but major artery; it is divided into three parts by the scalenus anterior muscle. The first, most medial part, has three branches:

- **internal thoracic** arteries, supplying the anterior intercostal spaces, diaphragm and anterior abdominal wall (p. 56)
- **vertebral** arteries, supplying the brain and spinal cord (p. 138)
- **thyrocervical trunk,** supplying the inferior thyroid and the scapular region (p. 36).

The branches of the second part (behind scalenus) and the third part (continues as the axillary artery) are variable; they usually include the costocervical trunk, which supplies the posterior part of the superior intercostal spaces, and the dorsal scapular artery, which contributes to the scapular anastomosis (p. 36).

🔍 ROOT OF THE NECK

The subclavian artery and lower trunk of the brachial plexus lie between the attachments of scalenus anterior and medius. They can be compressed by the tendons, causing symptoms in the limb; this is one of the causes of **thoracic outlet syndrome**.

Injuries in the root of the neck may cause a pneumothorax, damage to the brachial plexus or division of CN IX, causing paralysis of the trapezius.

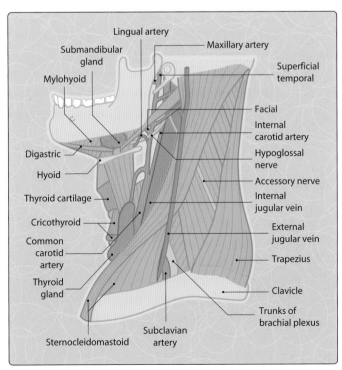

Fig. 3.65.3 Lateral view of the neck to show the posterior triangle.

66. The anterior triangle, thyroid gland and cervical lymph nodes

Questions
- At what level does the thyroid isthmus lie?
- Which nerve lies in the groove between the oesophagus and trachea?
- What is the connection between the foramen caecum of the tongue and the thyroid gland?

The major visceral components of the neck are the midline structures that make up the airway and the food passage together with the thyroid gland and the neurovascular bundles on either side.

Anterior triangles

Boundaries
The boundaries are (Figs 3.66.1 and 3.66.2):
- anterior border of sternocleidomastoid
- midline
- lower border of the mandible.

Contents
The contents of the anterior triangle are:
- **infrahyoid strap muscles,** which fix the position of the hyoid bone; they are the sternothyroid, sternohyoid, thyrohyoid and

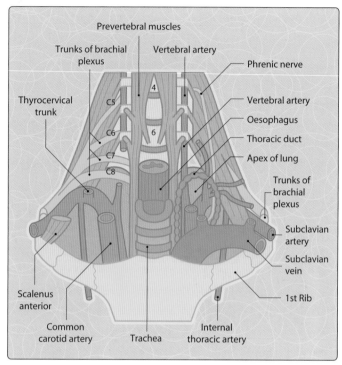

Fig. 3.66.2 Root of the neck with the clavicles and sternocleidomastoid removed.

omohyoid (their names give their attachments but in this case the thyroid means the cartilage not the gland) and they are supplied by C_1–C_3 via the **anser cervicalis** (Fig. 3.65.3, p. 155)
- **larynx** and its continuation, the **trachea**, below the cricoid cartilage at C6; the trachea ends at the sternal angle by dividing in two principal bronchi; it consists of C-shaped cartilages linked by elastic membranes and it can be palpated in the midline superior to the jugular notch
- **pharynx** and its continuation, the **oesophagus**, at C6; the oesophagus lies slightly to the left of the trachea
- **carotid sheath and its contents** (p. 154): at the level of the upper border of the thyroid cartilage, the common carotid artery divides into the internal and external carotid arteries; the vagus nerve lies between the internal carotid artery medially and the internal jugular vein laterally
- **lymph nodes**, many of which are palpable in this region, generally drain to the nearest nodes and eventually to the deep cervical chain; the tonsillar node lies just behind the angle of the mandible.

Lymph is returned to the venous system at the junction of the subclavian and internal jugular veins via the thoracic duct on the left (Fig. 3.66.3).

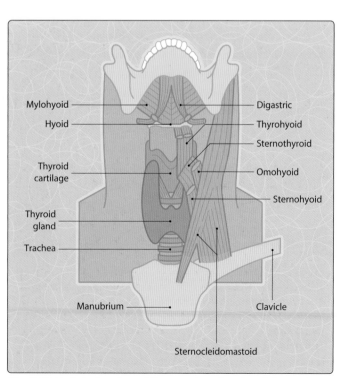

Fig. 3.66.1 Anterior view of the anterior triangles of the neck showing the strap muscles and thyroid gland.

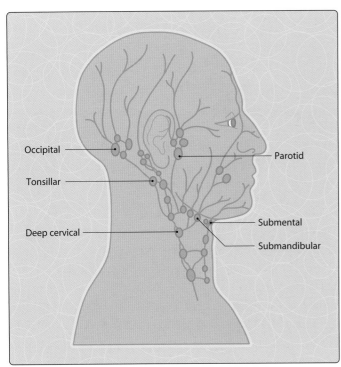

Fig. 3.66.3 Lateral view to show the major groups of lymph nodes in the neck.

Thyroid gland

The thyroid is an endocrine gland that secretes the thyroid hormones (thyroxine and triiodothyronine) and calcitonin. It consists of two lobes lying on either side of the trachea, linked anteriorly by the isthmus that lies in front of tracheal rings 2–4. It is bound to the trachea by the pretracheal fascia (p. 154). The superior part of the lobes is restricted by the attachment of sternothyroid to the thyroid cartilage; consequently, swellings of the gland (goitre) tend to expand inferiorly.

The boundaries are

- lateral surface under the sternothyroid and sternohyoid
- medial surface on either side of the larynx and trachea as far as the 6th tracheal ring
- posterior surface overlaps the carotid sheath.

Arterial and nerve supply

The arterial supply is a rich anastomosis derived from the superior thyroid artery (external carotid) and inferior thyroid artery (thyrocervical trunk of the subclavian). In a small proportion of the population there is an additional supply from the thyroid artery, which is a persistent embryonic vessel. It is a single vessel that ascends within the superior mediastinum and root of neck to the inferior margin of the thyroid. It may originate from the brachiocephalic trunk, arch of aorta or left common carotid artery.

The superior and middle thyroid veins drain to the internal jugular vein; inferiorly veins drain to the brachiocephalic veins.

Laryngeal nerves

The laryngeal nerves (branch of CN X) are closely related to blood supply to the thyroid. They are vulnerable to damage in thyroid surgery; damage results in paralysis of the laryngeal muscles (recurrent) and loss of sensory supply to the laryngeal inlet (superior). The vagus divides to give the **superior laryngeal nerve**, which divides again into the internal and external laryngeal nerves (Fig. 3.64.2A). The **external laryngeal nerve** passes inferiorly accompanied by the superior thyroid artery (a branch of the external carotid); it supplies a single laryngeal muscle. The **internal laryngeal nerve** supplies the mucous membrane of the larynx above the vocal folds.

At the root of the neck, the vagus nerve lies anterior to the subclavian artery as it passes through the thoracic inlet. At this level on the right, it branches to give the **right recurrent laryngeal nerve**, which hooks beneath the subclavian and passes superiorly to the larynx in a groove between the trachea and oesophagus (where it is closely related to the inferior thyroid artery). The **left recurrent laryngeal nerve** is a branch of the left vagus that arises close to the lung root in the thorax. It hooks beneath the arch of the aorta and travels superiorly in the groove between trachea and oesophagus with the left inferior thyroid artery. The recurrent laryngeal nerves supply all the remaining intrinsic muscles of the larynx and are sensory to the mucous membrane below the vocal folds.

Parathyroid glands

Two pairs of endocrine parathyroid glands (superior and inferior) lie embedded in the posterior surface of the thyroid; their positions are variable. The parathyroids secrete parathormone, which is involved in regulation of calcium levels in the blood.

 TWO SWELLINGS IN THE NECK ASSOCIATED WITH THE THYROID GLAND

Since the thyroid gland is attached to the trachea by pretracheal fascia, it moves upwards with the larynx and trachea during swallowing. If a patient is asked to swallow, any swelling of the thyroid will move upwards.

The thyroid develops as a downgrowth from the foramen caecum of the tongue. The thyroglossal duct marks the developmental track of thyroid tissue in the neck. Occasional, ectopic cells may give rise to thyroglossal cysts. In this case, a swelling resulting from a cyst will move when a patient sticks out the tongue.

67. Eye and ear

Questions
- Which cranial nerves are tested by the corneal reflex?
- Which division of the autonomic nervous system causes contraction of constrictor pupillae?
- What type of epithelium lines the tympanic membrane and middle ear cavity?

Eye

The eye is an outgrowth of the brain; the wall is composed of three coats (Fig. 3.67.1):

- outer: tough sclera is replaced anteriorly by the transparent cornea; there is a rich nerve supply from CN V_a (corneal reflex, p. 160)
- middle: vascular choroid replaced anteriorly by the ciliary body and iris
- inner: sensory retina.

The **anterior chamber** lies between cornea and iris and the **posterior chamber** between the iris and lens. The **ciliary body** secretes aqueous humour, which passes through the pupil to the anterior chamber where is it resorbed via the sinus venosus sclerae. Blockage can cause dangerous increase in intraocular pressure, leading to glaucoma. The **iris** comprises radially arranged smooth muscle (**dilator pupillae;** sympathetic control) and circular smooth muscle (**constrictor pupillae;** parasympathetic control via CN III and the ciliary ganglion).

The **ciliary processes** are radially arranged smooth muscle that allows accommodation of the lens (parasympathetic). The **lens** lies behind the pupil enclosed in a delicate capsule suspended from the ciliary processes by the suspensory ligament. Behind the lens the eye is filled with vitreous humour.

Retina

The outer layer of the retina is reflective (causes 'red eye' in flash photographs) and pigmented. The *deepest* layer of cells consists of light-sensitive **rods** and **cones.** These excite bipolar cells that synapse with ganglion cells. The axons pass backwards on the surface of the retina to form the optic nerve at the **optic disc.** The disc is also the blind spot where branches of the ophthalmic vessels enter and leave the eyeball in the centre of the optic nerve. The **fovea centralis** is the most light-sensitive area of the retina and is found 4 mm lateral to the optic disc. The extra-ocular muscles position the eye so that light from an object in view falls on the fovea.

Optic nerve

The optic nerve is covered by the meninges as is passes posteriorly in the optic canal to the middle cranial fossa and the optic chiasma. The central artery of the retina and its vein lie within the substance of the optic nerve where it enters the back of the eyeball. For part of their course, the vessels travel in the subarachnoid space, where the vein may be occluded if there is a rise in intracranial pressure. Increase in intracranial pressure can be detected as changes in the optic disc as viewed with an ophthalmoscope. The central artery is an 'end artery' and occlusion results in immediate and irreversible blindness.

Ear

The ear has complicated evolutionary and developmental origins. Its relations are very complex and only the simplest description can be given here. It has outer, middle and inner portions (Fig. 3.67.2).

Outer ear

The outer ear is routinely examined with an otoscope (Fig. 3.67.3). It consists of:

- the **pinna** (or auricle) with a skeleton of elastic cartilage
- the **external acoustic meatus,** which is one-third cartilage and two-thirds bony canal lined by a delicate epithelium that secretes protective wax (cerumen)
- the **tympanic membrane,** which completely separates the outer and middle ears, is a shallow cone with the apex

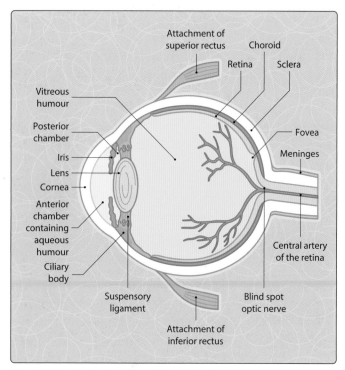

Fig. 3.67.1 Sagittal section of the eyeball.

Attachment of superior rectus
Choroid
Retina
Sclera
Vitreous humour
Posterior chamber
Fovea
Iris
Meninges
Lens
Cornea
Anterior chamber containing aqueous humour
Ciliary body
Central artery of the retina
Suspensory ligament
Blind spot optic nerve
Attachment of inferior rectus

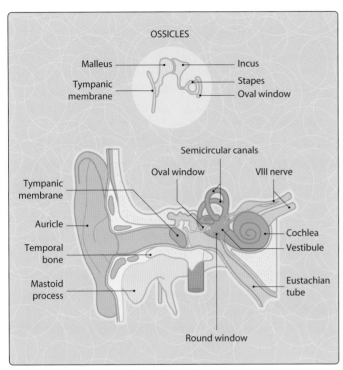

Fig. 3.67.2 The external, middle and inner ear.

embedded in the tympanic membrane and is visible with an otoscope (Fig. 3.67.3). There are four walls, roof and floor:

- lateral wall: tympanic membrane
- anterior wall: opening of the Eustachian tube leading down to the nasopharynx (Fig. 3.63.5)
- medial wall: bulge caused by the cochlea and oval window for the stapes; the facial nerve passes backwards and downwards in a bony canal, covered only by a delicate bony partition
- posterior wall: extends into the mastoid air cells
- inferiorly: the thin bony floor separates the middle ear from the internal carotid artery and internal jugular vein
- roof: part of the middle cranial fossa.

Because of the intimate relations of the middle ear, infections can cause confusing symptoms.

Inner ear

The inner ear is a closed hydraulic system (membranous labyrinth) entirely encased within the petrous temporal bone (bony labyrinth) (Fig. 3.67.4). It is concerned with the senses of hearing and balance (CN VIII).

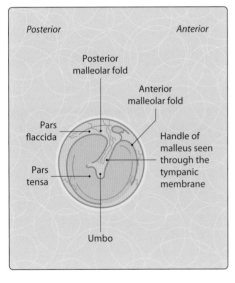

Fig. 3.67.3 Lateral view of the tympanic membrane as seen through an otoscope.

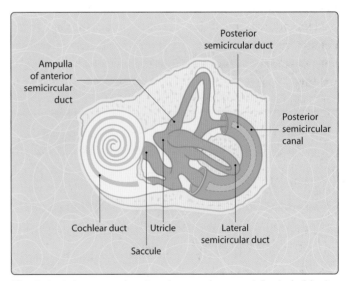

Fig. 3.67.4 Inner ear showing the membranous labyrinth (blue).

(umbo) pointing medially; it comprises three layers: skin, connective tissue, and an inner lining of *respiratory* epithelium (innervated by CN IX).

The sensory innervation of the outer ear is anteriorly by CN V$_c$ and posteriorly by CN X.

Middle ear

The middle ear or tympanic cavity is narrow from side to side. The ossicles (malleus, incus and stapes) span the superior part of the space and transmit sound vibrations between the tympanic membrane and the inner ear. The handle of the **malleus** is

---

REFERRED PAIN TO THE EAR

The anterior wall of the external auditory meatus and anterior part of the tympanic membrane are supplied by the auriculotemporal branch of CN V$_c$. The vagus nerve supplies the remainder. Disease of any structures supplied by the mandibular or vagus nerves may give rise to ear ache (referred pain, e.g. from the larynx, pharynx, tongue).

68. Clinical notes and testing of cranial nerves

Question
■ Can you list the tests for each of the cranial nerves I–XII?

I: olfactory nerve

Anosmia may be caused by head injuries that fracture the cribriform plate. It is also part of the normal ageing process. *Test*: patients will report loss of sense of smell.

II: optic nerve

Like CN I, the optic nerves are extensions of the brain. Within the optic canals, the optic nerves are surrounded by the meninges. At the optic chiasm, fibres from the nasal side of the visual field cross over (decussate) to the contralateral side. This results in the formation of the optic tracts, which then pass to the geniculate bodies of the thalamus. The axons finally relay in the visual cortex of the occipital lobes. Damage to CN II leads to complex symptoms, depending on the level of damage.

Tests:

■ **visual acuity:** eye charts
■ **visual fields:** can the patient follow a moving finger
■ **fundi:** examination with an ophthalmoscope.

III: oculomotor nerve

In addition to motor fibres, the oculomotor nerve carries para-sympathetic supply for pupilloconstriction *and* accommodation. Because it is closely related to the tentorial notch of the dura, this nerve is the first to show effects of traction in raised intracranial pressure. Damage to the nerve causes drooping of the eyelid (ptosis), lateral squint, dilatation of the pupil and loss of the accommodation reflex.

Tests:

■ visual light reflexes: tests both II and III
■ pupillary reflex: light shone into one eye causes constriction of both; it does not involve cerebral cortex activity and will occur in an unconscious patient – no response to light (i.e. fixed dilated pupils) indicates brain death
■ accommodation reflex: pupils should constrict then dilate if the patient focuses first on a near object and then looks away.

IV: trochlear nerve

CN IV arises from the dorsal surface of the midbrain; it has the longest intracranial course and is, therefore, vulnerable to raised intracranial pressure. Damage results in the eye turning medially and the patient complains of diplopia (double vision).

Test: the patient is asked to follow movements of a finger (adduction then depression).

V: trigeminal nerve

The trigeminal nerve has three divisions: V_a (**ophthalmic**), V_b (**maxillary**) and V_c (**mandibular**). Trigeminal neuralgia is severe pain over the sensory distribution of the branches of CN V. Shingles is caused by the *herpes zoster virus*, which may lie in the sensory ganglion of V and can cause a painful condition over the sensory distribution of one of the trigeminal divisions. The cornea may be involved if the ophthalmic division is affected. For the purposes of dental anaesthesia of the lower jaw, the inferior alveolar branch of the mandibular division is readily accessible from within the oral cavity (inferior alveolar nerve block). By contrast, the superior alveolar nerves must be infiltrated by injecting around the roots of individual teeth.

Test V_a:

■ touch on the skin of the forehead and scalp
■ lightly touching the cornea causes blinking (corneal reflex); this also tests CN VII.

Test V_b:

■ touch the skin of the lower eyelid, cheek and upper lip.

Test V_c:

■ touch the skin of the chin
■ look for contraction of masseter and temporalis muscles and the ability to open the mouth against resistance; the jaw deviates towards the side of the lesion when the patient opens their mouth.

VI: abducent nerve

The abducent nerve is vulnerable to raised intracranial pressure. The patient complains of diplopia and the eye is fully adducted, causing a medial squint.

Test: asking the patient to look to one side tests the medial rectus of one side (CN III) and lateral rectus of the other (CN VI).

VII: facial nerve

Of the motor cranial nerves, the facial nerve is the most commonly paralysed. The motor root and the nervus intermedius fibres lie within a bony canal, which is closely related to the inner ear and middle ear cavity. The terminal parts of its motor branches lie within the substance of the parotid gland. The facial nerve may be affected by diseases (or surgery) of any of these structures. Depending on the level of damage, injury may cause paralysis of the facial muscles (loss of blinking, drooping of the angle of the mouth) with loss of the sense of taste from the anterior two-thirds of the tongue and loss of secretion from the lacrimal and salivary glands. It is also vulnerable to damage during a forceps delivery of a baby because of the rudimentary development of the mastoid process in the newborn.

Tests:

■ look for facial symmetry (movements and skin creases)
■ corneal reflex (i.e. blinking; also tests CN V_a).

VIII: vestibulocochlear nerve

Damage to the nerve or blockage of the external and/or middle ear will cause unilateral hearing loss, tinnitus (noises in the ear) and vertigo (loss of balance).

Test: use vibration of a tuning fork to distinguish between conductive and sensorineural deafness.

IX: glossopharygeal nerve

The glossopharygeal nerve provides an important sensory supply to the posterior one-third of the tongue, the oropharynx, auditory tube and middle ear. It also provides a motor supply to the soft palate and pharynx. Damage can result in loss of sensation on the affected side and noticeable effects on swallowing.

Test: the gag reflex tests CN IX for sensation and CN X for motor response.

X: vagus nerve

The vagus nerve controls the voluntary muscles and gives a sensory supply to the larynx, pharynx and superior oesophagus and carries parasympathetic supply to thoracic and abdominal viscera. The recurrent laryngeal nerves that supply the larynx are at risk in thyroid surgery and hoarseness of the voice may be a symptom of malignancy either in the neck or thorax.

The normal position of the vocal folds as seen at laryngoscopy is illustrated in Fig. 3.68.1. Complete division of one of the recurrent laryngeal nerves causes the fold on the affected side to take up a neutral position, which is half way between the adducted and abducted position and speech is not greatly affected. If both nerves are divided, the voice is lost completely and breathing becomes difficult through the partially open glottis. However, if one of the nerves is only *partly* damaged, the affected vocal fold takes up the fully *add*ucted position because the abductor (posterior cricoarytenoid) is usually totally paralysed; it follows that the cords will be fully adducted in the midline following bilateral *partial* damage and a tracheostomy may become essential.

Tests:

■ normal speech and swallowing
■ gag reflex

■ observe movement of the soft palate when patient says 'aah': the uvula will deviate to the unaffected side.

XI: accessory nerve

Because it is nearly subcutaneous in the posterior triangle of the neck, CN XI is vulnerable to traumatic lacerations and also during biopsy of cervical lymph nodes and other procedures in the region. The cranial part of the accessory nerve contributes to the distribution of CN X and the spinal part supplies sterno-cleidomastoid and trapezius.

Tests:

■ ask the patient to turn their chin to one side (rotating to the right tests the left sternocleidomastoid muscle)
■ ask the patient to shrug their shoulders against resistance.

XII: hypoglossal nerve

Movements of the tongue are important in chewing, swallowing and speech. Division of the hypoglossal nerve results in paralysis, which causes the tongue to deviate to the ipsilateral side. After some time, wasting of muscles causes the tongue to appear shrunken and wrinkled.

In an unconscious casualty or an anaesthetized patient lying on their back, the tongue is effectively paralysed and will fall back into the pharynx, where it may block the airway. Because the root of the tongue is fixed to the hyoid and mandible, pulling the latter forward pulls the tongue forward and opens the airway.

Test: protrusion of the tongue (deviation to weak side suggests unilateral damage).

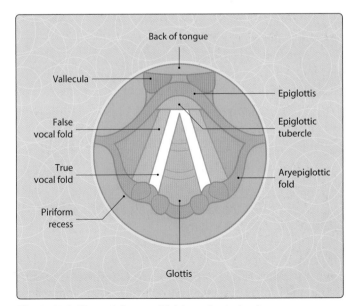

Fig. 3.68.1 View of the vocal folds as through a laryngoscope.

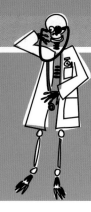

Glossary

Some hints on anatomical terminology

Anatomical and other medical terminology is based on an understanding of a relatively few basic elements. These elements are the roots, prefixes and suffixes that are used in various combinations to form many medical terms. They are commonly derived from Latin or Greek words. A root is the basic part of a word, for example gastro- refers to the stomach. A prefix may be added before the root to alter its meaning. An example of a prefix is epi- meaning on or above, which with the root gastro forms the word epigastric, meaning on or above the stomach. A suffix is a word ending. For example -itis means inflammation so that gastritis is inflammation of the stomach.

Other terms are compound words using two roots like cyto- meaning cell and -ology meaning study: cytology is the study of cells.

This glossary consists of commonly used anatomical terms with their meaning and some examples, as well as some useful roots, prefixes and suffixes. Plurals (pl.) and adjectives (adj.) are also given if they might cause confusion.

a-/an-
absent or deficient, e.g. anaemia

ab-
away from, e.g. abduction is movement away from midline

ad-
towards, e.g. adduction is movement towards midline

adrenal
endocrine gland located near the kidney (literally meaning towards the kidney); it is also called suprarenal gland (i.e. above the kidney)

afferent
carrying towards a given point; afferent nerve impulses (i.e. sensory) are carried towards the brain and spinal cord

agonist muscle
one that on contraction causes a specific movement (prime mover; e.g. biceps brachii causes flexion of the elbow); contraction of the agonist usually requires the relaxation of the antagonist; *see* antagonist

anastomosis
network of communicating arteries, veins or nerves (pl. anastomoses)

antagonist muscle
one that has the opposite action of a given movement, e.g. triceps is the antagonist to flexion of the elbow

anterior
front of a structure, equivalent to ventral (antero- in combinations)

apex
pointed end of a cone-shaped structure, e.g. apex of the lung (adj. apical)

aponeurosis
flattened tendon attaching across a wide area to bone

appendicular
relating to the appendages (i.e. the limbs), as in appendicular skeleton

arachnoid
middle layer of the meninges

arrector pili
smooth muscle attached to the base of hair follicles; contractions cause 'goose bumps'

arthro-
relates to joints, e.g. arthritis, arthroscope

atrium
the two smaller chambers of the heart (pl. atria, adj. atrial)

atrophy
wasting

autonomic nervous system (ANS)
controls involuntary activity of the body (e.g. heart rate, sweating); it is divided into sympathetic and para-sympathetic divisions

axial
relating to the axis of the body as in axial skeleton, which consists of the skull, vertebral column and thoracic cage

axilla
region where the upper limb joins the trunk, also armpit, e.g. axillary artery, axillary lymph nodes

axon
the fibre of a neuron(e), which conducts impulses away from the cell body

bifid/bifurcation
divided into two: spinous processes of the cervical vertebrae are bifid; the bifurcation of the trachea is a division into two, the right and left primary bronchi

biopsy
sample of tissue removed for histological examination

-blast
primitive cell or structure that gives rise to other cell types or structures, e.g. osteoblasts are primitive bone-forming cells; see also -cyte

brachial
relates to the arm (between the shoulder and elbow), hence brachial artery

branchial
a series of branchial arches (primitive gill arches) at the cranial end of the embryonic digestive system give rise to specific structures of the head and neck

bronchiole
microscopic branches of the bronchi

bronchus
first branches of the trachea (pl. bronchi, adj. bronchial)

buccal
relates to the mouth

bursa
small sac lined by synovial membrane that ensures free movement of tendons close to joints, e.g. infrapatellar bursa

bursitis
inflammation of a bursa

cancer
tumour that can spread to other tissues

carcinoma
cancer of epithelial (rather than connective tissue) origin (carcinogen is a cancer-causing substance)

cardia
heart (adj. cardiac)

caudal
towards or nearer to the sacrum, e.g. the kidneys are caudal to the diaphragm

central nervous system (CNS)
the part of the nervous system that includes the brain and spinal cord

cephalic
nearer to, or relating to, the head

cerebellum
part of the brain that controls coordinated movement, balance and muscle tone (adj. cerebellar)

cerebrum
largest part of the brain, comprising the cerebral hemi-spheres (adj. cerebral)

cerebrospinal fluid (CSF)
fluid that surrounds the CNS and fills the internal ventricles

cervix
the neck, also the narrow part or 'neck' of an organ, e.g. cervix of the uterus (adj. cervical)

colon
main part of the large intestine (adj. colic)

chondro-
relates to cartilage, e.g. chondrocytes are cartilage cells

collateral
a subsidiary or accessory structure (e.g. collateral branches of nerves and arteries); also side by side (e.g. lateral and medial ligaments of the knee)

computed tomography (CT)
an imaging method that uses X-rays to create cross-sectional views of the body; also CAT (computed axial tomography) scan

condyle
literally means knuckle; rounded articular surface, e.g. femoral condyles

coronal
side-to-side plane between the ears that divides the body into anterior and posterior parts

coronary
relating to the heart (Latin: *cor* is heart)

corpus
literally means body, e.g. corpus callosum, corpus luteum (pl. corpora)

cortex
outer part of a structure, e.g adrenal cortex (adj. cortical); *see also* medulla

costa
rib, e.g. intercostal muscles lie between the ribs (adj. costal)

cranium
bones that enclose the brain, e.g. cranial nerves; also means towards or nearer the head (adj. cranial)

crus
a structure that resembles a pair of legs, a pair of diverging limbs or bands, e.g. the crura of the diaphragm, penis and clitoris

cusp
leaflet of a valve; hence bicuspid valve means a valve comprising two leaflets

cutaneous
relates to the skin

-cyte or cyto-
cell or mature cell type, e.g. osteocyte is a mature bone cell and cytology is the study of cells; *see also* -blast

deep
far or further from the surface; *see* superficial

dental
related to teeth (dens is a tooth-shaped structure)

dermatome
an area of skin supplied by a single spinal segment

dermis
deep connective tissue layer of the skin; epidermis lies on (is superficial to) the dermis (adj. dermal)

diastole
relaxation phase of the cardiac cycle (adj. diastolic); *see* systole

distal
further away from the midline of the body or root of a structure, e.g. the hand is distal to the elbow; *see* proximal

dorsal
towards the back (with reference to anatomical position); similar to posterior in erect humans

dorsiflexion
bending the foot upwards at the ankle (opposite is plantarflexion)

duodenum
first part of the small intestine

dura
outer tough layer of the meninges (dura mater)

-ectomy
surgical removal, e.g. tonsillectomy is removal of the tonsils

efferent
carrying away from, e.g. efferent (i.e. motor) nerve impulses are carried away from the CNS

endo-
on the inside; e.g. endothelium is the lining of blood vessels, endometrium lines the uterus, endoscope is a telescope for looking inside the body

endocrine
secretion by a cell (or gland) directly into the bloodstream; *see* exocrine

embryo
developing offspring during the first 2 months of pregnancy (adj. embryonic)

epi-
above or on the surface of a structure, e.g. epidermis is the outermost layer of the skin, epigastric relates to the area of the abdomen just below the sternum (literally means on the belly), epicondyle projection is on or above a condyle

epithelium
one of the four basic tissue types; it forms glands, covers all surfaces and lines the body cavities (adj. epithelial)

eversion
turning the sole of the foot outwards (laterally)

ex- extra-
out, e.g. expiration is to breathe out, extracapsular is the outside of a joint capsule

exocrine
secretion by a cell or group of cells into a duct for transport elsewhere (*see* endocrine)

extend
usually means to straighten a joint (*see* flexion); extensor muscles increase the angle between the bones at a joint

extrinsic
a structure that begins outside the area it acts upon (e.g. the extrinsic muscles of the hand such as flexor digitorum superficialis arise in the forearm)

fascia
connective tissue; superficial fascia is loose connective tissue found immediately beneath the skin; deep fascia forms fairly tough sheets or sheaths around muscles and neurovascular bundles, e.g. carotid sheath

fetus/foetus
offspring from the third month of pregnancy (adj. fetal)

fibular
lateral side of the leg (also alternative for peroneal)

flex
usually means to fold a joint; flexor muscles decrease the angle between the bones at a joint; see extension

foramen
opening or passage through a bone, e.g. foramen magnum through which the spinal cord passes (pl. foramina)

fornix
literally means an arch; prostitutes frequented the arches of the colosseum in ancient Rome, hence the word fornication (pl. fornices)

fossa
literally means a ditch, so is a depression, hollow or pit (pl. fossae)

fovea
depression or pit

frontal
relates to the forehead or to the anterior part of an organ

fundus
base of a hollow organ or the part furthest from the opening (stomach, uterus)

ganglion
a swelling; in the nervous system; it is a collection of nerve cell bodies outside the CNS, e.g. a sensory ganglion or an autonomic ganglion; see nucleus

gastr- gastro-
relates to the belly or gastrum, which usually means the stomach, e.g. gastric artery, gastrointestinal (GI) tract, gastroscopy

gastrocnemius
muscle of the calf that flexes the knee and plantar flexes the ankle

glosso-
relates to the tongue; the hypoglossal nerve lies below the tongue

glottis
gap between the vocal folds (adj. glottal)

gonads
sex organs: female ovaries and male testes (adj. gonadal)

gyrus
raised area of the cerebral cortex (pl. gyri); see sulcus

haemo- (US: hemo-)
relates to blood, e.g. haematology is the study of blood; haematoma (bruising) swelling is caused by bleeding into the tissues

hepato-
relates to the liver, e.g. hepatic artery; hepatitis is inflammation of the liver

hernia
protrusion of an organ or tissue through the wall of a cavity that normally encloses it, e.g. femoral and inguinal hernias

hiatus
gap, opening

hilum
place where vessels and nerves enter or leave an organ, e.g. hilum of the lung (adj. hilar)

homo
literally staying the same, e.g. homeostasis is maintenance of the body within fixed limits

homologous
having the same origin (often developmental origin)

hyper-
literally above, or excessive, e.g. hyperextension is forced extension of a joint beyond normal limits; hypertrophy is increase in size

hypo-
literally below or depressed, e.g. hypochondrium is below the costal cartilages, hypoglossal is below the tongue

ileum
last part of the small intestine, e.g. iliocolic junction

ilium
makes up the hip bone with the pubis and ischium (adj. iliac)

inferior
below or lower, e.g. inferior vena cava drains the lower part of the body

infra-
below or lower, e.g. infraorbital is below the orbit of the skull, infrahyoid is below the hyoid, infracolic is below the colon in the abdomen bone

infundibulum
narrow or funnel-shaped region, e.g. infundibulum of the pituitary or the uterine tube

inguinal
relates to the groin where the lower limb meets the trunk, e.g. inguinal hernia

insertion
relates to the more distal attachment of a muscle which moves on contraction of the muscle

inter-
between, e.g. interosseous membrane lies between the bones, intercostal between the ribs

intra-
inside, e.g. intracranial is inside the cranium, an intra-capsular tendon lies inside the capsule of the joint; *see* extra-

intrinsic
a muscle or ligament that begins within the structure it acts upon, e.g. the intrinsic muscles of the hand arise and insert within the hand

invagination
vagina means a sheath, invaginate means to push one structure or layer inside another, e.g. the lung is invaginated into the pleural membrane

inversion
turning the sole of the foot inwards (medially) at the subtalar joint complex

ipsilateral
on the same side (opposite side is contralateral)

ischioanal/ischiorectal
synonymous terms

isthmus
narrow region connecting two parts, e.g. isthmus of the thyroid gland

-itis
inflammation, e.g. gastritis is inflammation of the stomach, arthritis is inflammation of joint

jejunum
second part of the small intestine (adj. jejunal)

labium
lip (pl. labia, adj. labial)

laparo-
relates to the abdomen, e.g. laparoscopy looks inside the abdomen, laparotomy is opening the abdomen

larynx
that part of the airway between pharynx and trachea; contains the vocal cords, e.g. in laryngoscope, laryngitis (adj. laryngeal)

lateral
further from the midline towards the side, *see* medial

ligament
tough connective tissue bands that tie together two or more structures, most commonly bones (adj. ligamentous)

lingula
tongue (adj. lingual)

lumen
central cavity of a tube, e.g. artery, vein, intestine, etc. (adj. luminal)

macro-
large

magnetic resonance imaging (MRI)
a non-invasive, non-X-ray imaging technique that depends upon the detection of the movement of hydrogen atoms in response to radiowaves in a powerful magnetic field

mast-
relating to the breast, e.g. mastectomy is removal of the breast, mastitis is inflammation of the breast

meatus
pathway or passage, e.g. external auditory meatus (ear hole)

medial
nearer the midline; *see* lateral

median
in the midline

meninges
three connective tissue layers (pia, arachnoid and dura) that surround the CNS (adj. meningeal)

medulla
inner part of a solid organ, e.g. medulla of the kidney (adj. medullary); *see* cortex

mesentery
double layer of peritoneum that attaches viscera to the posterior abdominal wall (adj. mesenteric)

metro-
relating to the uterus, e.g. myometrium is uterine muscle, endometrium is uterine lining

mitral
relates to the valve between the left atrium and left ventricle (left atrioventricular valve, bicuspid valve)

motor
relates to structures or activities that involve transmitting nerve impulses away from the CNS; *see also* efferent

mucus
sticky liquid produced by glands (adj. mucous)

myo-
relating to muscle, e.g. myocardium is muscle of the heart, myometrium is uterine muscle, myalgia is muscle pain

nerve
strictly it should refer to a large collection of nerve fibres that can be seen with the naked eye (e.g. the ulnar nerve) but it may also refer to a single neurone or its axon; it is a term that may be used rather loosely

neuro-
relates to nerves, e.g. neurology is study of the nervous system

nucleus
in terms of the CNS, a nucleus is a collection of nerve cell bodies that share a similar function; *see also* ganglion

omentum
folds of peritoneum that link the stomach to other viscera, e.g. lesser omentum connects the stomach to the liver

os- osteo-
relates to bones, e.g. ossification process of bone formation, osteoporosis is abnormal loss of bone density

-oma
denotes a tumour, e.g. lymphoma (of the lymph nodes), carcinoma (of an epithelium)

-ostomy
making a permanent opening, e.g. tracheostomy is a permanent (or semipermanent) opening into the trachea

-otomy
making a small, temporary opening, e.g. laryngotomy is an emergency opening into the larynx

palpation
examination of the body by feeling with the fingers (adj. palpable)

palpebra
the eyelids, e.g. the muscle that lifts the eyelids is levator palpebrae superior (pl. palpebrae, adj. palpebral)

para-
by the side of, e.g. paravertebral is alongside the vertebral column, para-aortic is beside the aorta

parietal
relates to the inner walls of a body cavity, e.g. parietal pleura; also relates to the parietal bone of the skull

path-
relates to disease, e.g. pathology

peri-
around or near, e.g. periosteum is the membrane covering the surface of bone

perineal
relates to the perineum, the area between the thighs (not to be confused with peroneal)

peroneal
relates to the lateral side of the leg (alternative for fibular)

phrenic
relates to the diaphragm

pia
inner vascular layer of the meninges

plexus
network of branching structures, e.g. brachial plexus is the network of nerves that supply the upper limb

portal system
venous system that carries blood through a second capillary bed before returning blood to the heart, e.g. hepatic portal vein delivers blood from the GI tract to the capillaries of the liver before it is returned to the right atrium via the hepatic vein and the inferior vena cava

posterior
towards the back; *see also* dorsal

proprioception
ability to sense of the position of the body in space; proprioceptors are present in muscles and tendons and register mechanical changes in position

prone
patient lying face down

proximal
nearer to the midline of the body or the root of a structure, e.g. the elbow is proximal to the hand; *see also* distal

pulmonary circulation
vessels that carry blood from the right side of the heart to the alveolar capillaries of the lungs and back to the left side of the heart; in the process gaseous exchange occurs with oxygen entering the blood and carbon dioxide leaving it

radial
lateral side of the forearm or hand

ramus
branch (pl. rami)

raphe
literally a seam; line of union between two muscles such as is found in the pharyngeal constrictors

renal
relating to the kidneys, e.g. renal artery

retro-
behind, e.g. retroperitoneal behind the peritoneum

sagittal
a plane that divides the body or structure into right and left portions

sensory
relates to structures or activities that involve transmitting nerve impulses towards the CNS from the periphery, *see also* afferent

serous
thin, watery secretion such as is secreted by a serous membrane like the pleura; *see* mucous

sinus
cavity or channel

somatic
relates to the structures that make up the body wall or its primitive divisions, known as somites

sphincter
muscular valve that controls the diameter of a tube, e.g. the pyloric sphincter lies between the stomach and duodenum

splanchnic
equivalent to visceral (splanchnic is derived from Greek, visceral from Latin)

squamous
flattened, scale-like cells, e.g. squamous epithelium consists of very flattened cells

sulcus
gutter or depression; particularly used in relation to the surface of the cerebrum where sulci lie between the gyri (pl. sulci)

superficial
near, or nearer, the surface; *see* deep

supine
patient lying on their back, face up

supra-
above, e.g. supraorbital nerve; supracolic is above the colon in the abdomen

superior
above, e.g. superior vena cava drains the blood from the upper part of the body

synapse
junction between two neurones or between a nerve and an effector

synovial
freely movable joints; literally synovial means like an egg; synovial fluid secreted by the synovial membrane has the consistency of egg white and lubricates and nourishes the joint surfaces

systemic circulation
vessels that carry blood from the left side of the heart to the capillary beds of the entire body (except the lungs) and back to the right side of the heart; in the process gaseous exchange occurs with oxygen leaving the blood and carbon dioxide entering it

systole
contraction phase of the cardiac cycle (adj. systolic); *see also* diastole

tendon
the tough extension of the connective tissue associated with muscles that forms the attachment of muscle to bone

thoraco-
relating to the thorax

tibial
medial side of the leg

tissue
similar cells that perform specialized functions; there are four basic types: epithelia, muscle, nerve and connective tissues

transverse
a plane that divides a structure into superior and inferior parts

trochlea
a pulley or a structure shaped like a pulley

ulnar
medial side of the forearm or hand

ureter
the muscular tube that carries urine between the kidney and the bladder

urethra
the muscular tube that carries urine from the bladder to the exterior

varicose
enlarged and twisted superficial veins, especially in the lower limb

vaso-
relating to vessels, e.g. vasoconstriction; physiological narrowing of blood vessels

ventral
towards the front and equivalent to anterior in the anatomical position

ventricle
chamber, e.g. thicker-walled chambers of the heart; there are also four ventricles in the brain

vesical
relates to the bladder

visceral
relates to internal organs; visceral nerves tend to be under involuntary control and sensation tends to be vague and imprecisely perceptible or even imperceptible; see also somatic

viscus
internal organ, e.g. heart, spleen, etc. (pl. viscera)

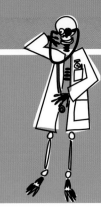

Index